Best Practices

for Comprehensive Tobacco Control Programs

2014

The following individuals from the
Centers for Disease Control and Prevention,
National Center for Chronic Disease Prevention and Health Promotion,
Office on Smoking and Health (OSH),
were primary contributors to the preparation of this publication:

Brian King, PhD, MPH
Terry Pechacek, PhD
Peter Mariolis, PhD

**The following OSH staff
also contributed to the preparation of this publication:**

Judy Ahearn, BS; Stephen Babb, MPH; Diane Beistle, BA; Rebecca Bunnell, PhD; Ralph Caraballo, PhD; Shanta Dube, PhD, MPH; Monica Eischen, BS; Jami Fraze, PhD; Erika Fulmer, MHA; Bridgette Garrett, PhD, MS; Karen Gutierrez, BA; Carissa Holmes, MPH; David Homa, PhD, MPH; Brandon Kenemer, MPH; Rene Lavinghouze, MA; Allison MacNeil, MPH; Ann Malarcher, PhD, MSPH; Kristy Marynak, MPP; Timothy A. McAfee, MD, MPH; Sarah O'Leary, MPH, MA; Gabbi Promoff, MA; Robert Rodes, MS, MBA, MEd; Patti Seikus, MPH; Shawna Shields, MPH; Kisha Smith, MPH; Karla S. Sneegas, MPH; Xin Xu, PhD; and Lei Zhang, PhD.

**OSH also gratefully acknowledges
the contributions provided by the following individuals:**

David Abrams, PhD, Legacy; Rob Adsit, MEd, University of Wisconsin; Linda Bailey, MHS, JD, North American Quitline Consortium; Cathy Callaway, BS, American Cancer Society Cancer Action Network; Jennifer Cantrell, DrPH, MPA, Legacy; Thomas Carr, BA, American Lung Association; Julia Cartwright, BA, Legacy; Frank Chaloupka, PhD, University of Illinois–Chicago; K. Michael Cummings, PhD, MPH, Medical University of South Carolina; Marietta Dreher, BA, ClearWay Minnesota; Sherry Emery, PhD, MBA, University of Illinois–Chicago; Matthew Farrelly, PhD, RTI International; John Francis, MPH, MBA, CDC's Division of Community Health; Karen Girard, MPA, Oregon Healthy Authority; Emma Goforth, MPH, Colorado Department of Public Health and Environment; Roy Hart, MPH, Mississippi State Department of Health; Sally Herndon, MPH, North Carolina Division of Public Health; Delmonte Jefferson, National African American Tobacco Prevention Network; Harlan Juster, PhD, New York State Department of Health; Pamela Ling, MD, MPH, University of California at San Francisco; Doug Luke, PhD, Washington University–St. Louis; Marc Manley, MD, MPH, University of Pittsburg Medical Center; Danny McGoldrick, PhD, Campaign for Tobacco-Free Kids; Jeannette Noltenius, PhD, MA, National Latino Tobacco Control Network; Sjonna Paulson, APR, Oklahoma Tobacco Settlement Endowment; Meg Riordan, PhD, Campaign for Tobacco-Free Kids; Todd Rogers, PhD, RTI International; April Roeseler, MSPH, BSN, California Department of Public Health; Mary Kate Salley, BA, Alere Wellbeing; Scout, PhD, National LGBT Tobacco Control Network; Chris Sherwin, BA, American Heart Association; Jennifer Singleterry, MA, American Lung Association; Madeline Solomon, MPH, Tobacco Technical Assistance Consortium; Jeff Soukup, BS, Nebraska Department of Health and Human Services; Colleen Stevens, MS, California Department of Public Health; Bob Vollinger, MSPH, National Cancer Institute; Donna Warner, MBA, MA, Multi-State Collaborative for Health Systems Change to Address Tobacco Use; Jeff Willett, PhD, Kansas Health Foundation; and David Willoughby, MA, ClearWay Minnesota.

Table of Contents

Executive Summary 6

Introduction 9

Section A: Components of a Comprehensive Tobacco Control Program 17

    I. State and Community Interventions 18

    II. Mass-Reach Health
Communication Interventions 30

    III. Cessation Interventions 40

    IV. Surveillance and Evaluation 56

    V. Infrastructure, Administration, and Management 64

Section B: Recommended Funding Levels for All 50 States and the District Of Columbia 71

    Annual Total Funding Levels for State Programs 72

    Annual Per Capita Funding Levels for State Programs 74

Section C: Recommended Funding Levels, by State 77

Appendices 129

    Appendix A: Funding Recommendation Formulations 130

    Appendix B: Program and Policy Recommendations for
Comprehensive Tobacco Control Programs 133

    Appendix C: National Prevention Strategy Recommendations 136

    Appendix D: Guidelines for Comprehensive Local Tobacco Control Programs 138

    Appendix E: Data Sources 139

Executive Summary

Tobacco use is the single most preventable cause of disease, disability, and death in the United States. Nearly one-half million Americans still die prematurely from tobacco use each year, and more than 16 million Americans suffer from a disease caused by smoking. Despite these risks, approximately 42.1 million U.S. adults currently smoke cigarettes. And the harmful effects of smoking do not end with the smoker. Secondhand smoke exposure causes serious disease and death, and even brief exposure can be harmful to health. Each year, primarily because of exposure to secondhand smoke, an estimated 7,330 nonsmoking Americans die of lung cancer and more than 33,900 die of heart disease. Coupled with this enormous health toll is the significant economic burden. Economic costs attributable to smoking and exposure to secondhand smoke now approach $300 billion annually.

Fifty years have passed since the 1964 Surgeon General's report on smoking and health concluded: "Cigarette smoking is a health hazard of sufficient importance in the United States to warrant appropriate remedial action." There now is a robust evidence base for effective tobacco control interventions. Yet, despite this progress, the United States is not currently on track to achieve the *Healthy People 2020* objective to reduce cigarette smoking among adults to 12% or less by the year 2020. A 2007 Institute of Medicine (IOM) report presented a blueprint for action to "reduce smoking so substantially that it is no longer a public health problem for our nation." The two-pronged strategy for achieving this goal includes: 1) strengthening and fully implementing currently proven tobacco control measures; and 2) changing the regulatory landscape to permit policy innovations. Foremost among the IOM recommendations is that each state should fund a comprehensive tobacco control program at the level that the Centers for Disease Control and Prevention (CDC) recommends.

Evidence-based, statewide tobacco control programs that are comprehensive, sustained, and accountable have been shown to reduce smoking rates, as well as tobacco-related diseases and deaths. A comprehensive statewide tobacco control program is a coordinated effort to establish smokefree policies and social norms, to promote and assist tobacco users to quit, and to prevent initiation of tobacco use. This comprehensive approach combines educational, clinical, regulatory, economic, and social strategies. Research has documented the effectiveness of laws and policies in a comprehensive tobacco control effort to protect the public from secondhand smoke exposure, promote cessation, and prevent initiation, including: increasing the unit price of tobacco products; implementing comprehensive smokefree laws that prohibit smoking in all indoor areas of worksites, restaurants, and bars, and encouraging smokefree private settings such as multiunit housing; providing insurance coverage of evidence-based tobacco cessation treatments; and limiting minors' access to tobacco products. Additionally, research has shown greater effectiveness with multicomponent interventional efforts that integrate the implementation of programmatic and policy initiatives to influence social norms, systems, and networks.

CDC's *Best Practices for Comprehensive Tobacco Control Programs—2014* is an evidence-based guide to help states plan and establish comprehensive tobacco control programs. This edition updates *Best Practices for Comprehensive Tobacco Control Programs—2007*. The 2014 edition describes an integrated programmatic structure for implementing interventions proven to be effective and provides the recommended level of state investment to reach these goals and to reduce tobacco use in each state.

These individual components are most effective when they work together to produce the synergistic effects of a comprehensive statewide tobacco control program. On the basis of evidence of effectiveness documented in the scientific literature and the experiences of state and local programs, the most effective population-based approaches have been defined within the following overarching components.

Executive Summary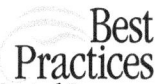

I. State and Community Interventions

State and community interventions include supporting and implementing programs and policies to influence societal organizations, systems, and networks that encourage and support individuals to make behavior choices consistent with tobacco-free norms. The social norm change model presumes that lasting change occurs through shifts in the social environment — initially or ultimately — at the grassroots level across local communities. State and community interventions unite a range of integrated activities, including local and statewide policies and programs, as well as initiatives to eliminate tobacco-related disparities.

The most effective state and community interventions are those in which specific strategies for promoting tobacco use cessation, preventing tobacco use initiation, and eliminating exposure to secondhand smoke are combined with mass-reach health communication interventions and other initiatives to mobilize communities and to integrate these strategies into synergistic and multicomponent efforts.

II. Mass-Reach Health Communication Interventions

An effective state-level, mass-reach health communication intervention delivers strategic, culturally appropriate, and high-impact messages through sustained and adequately funded campaigns that are integrated into a comprehensive state tobacco control program. Typically, effective health communication interventions and countermarketing strategies employ a wide range of paid and earned media, including: television, radio, out-of-home (e.g., billboards, transit), print, and digital advertising at the state and local levels; promotion through public relations/earned media efforts, including press releases/conferences, social media, and local events; health promotion activities, such as working with health care professionals and other partners, promoting quitlines, and offering free nicotine replacement therapy; and efforts to reduce or replace tobacco industry sponsorship and promotions.

Innovations in health communication interventions include the ability to target and engage specific audiences through multiple communication channels, such as online video, mobile Web, and smartphone and tablet applications (apps). Social media platforms, such as Twitter and Facebook, have facilitated improvements in how messages are developed, fostered, and disseminated in order to better communicate with target audiences and allow for relevant, credible messages to be shared more broadly within the target audiences' social circles.

III. Cessation Interventions

Comprehensive state tobacco control program cessation activities can focus on three broad goals: (1) promoting health systems change; (2) expanding insurance coverage of proven cessation treatments; and (3) supporting state quitline capacity.

Health systems change involves institutionalizing cessation interventions in health care systems and seamlessly integrating these interventions into routine clinical care. These actions increase the likelihood that health care providers will consistently screen patients for tobacco use and intervene with patients who use tobacco, thus increasing cessation. Expanding cessation insurance coverage removes cost and administrative barriers that prevent smokers from accessing cessation counseling and medications, and increases the number of smokers who use evidence-based cessation treatments and who successfully quit. Expanding cessation insurance coverage also has the potential to reduce tobacco-related population disparities.

Quitlines potentially have broad reach, are effective with and can be tailored to diverse populations, and increase quit rates. Because state quitline services are free, remove time and transportation barriers, and are confidential, they are one of the most accessible cessation resources. Optimally, quitline counseling should be made available to all tobacco users willing to access the service.

IV. Surveillance and Evaluation

Surveillance is the process of continuously monitoring attitudes, behaviors, and health outcomes over time. Statewide surveillance is important for monitoring the achievement of overall program goals. Evaluation is used to assess the implementation and outcomes of a program, increase efficiency and impact over time, and demonstrate accountability.

Publicly financed programs need to have accountability and demonstrate effectiveness, as well as have access to timely data that can be used for program improvement and decision making.

Therefore, a critical infrastructural component of any comprehensive tobacco control program is a surveillance and evaluation system that can monitor and document key short-term, intermediate, and long-term outcomes within populations. Data from surveillance and evaluation systems can be used to inform program and policy directions, demonstrate program effectiveness, monitor progress on reducing health disparities, ensure accountability to those with fiscal oversight, and engage stakeholders.

V. Infrastructure, Administration, and Management

A comprehensive tobacco control program requires considerable funding to implement. Therefore, a fully functioning infrastructure must be in place in order to achieve the capacity to implement effective interventions. Sufficient capacity is essential for program sustainability, efficacy, and efficiency, and it enables programs to plan their strategic efforts, provide strong leadership, and foster collaboration among the state and local tobacco control communities.

An adequate number of skilled staff is also necessary to provide or facilitate program oversight, technical assistance, and training.

The primary objectives of the recommended statewide comprehensive tobacco control program are to reduce tobacco use and the personal and societal burdens of tobacco-related disease and death. Research shows that the more states spend on comprehensive tobacco control programs, the greater the reductions in smoking. The longer states invest in such programs, the greater and quicker the impact.

Implementing comprehensive tobacco control programs at the levels of investment outlined in this report would have a substantial impact. As a result, millions of fewer people in the United States would smoke and hundreds of thousands of premature tobacco-related deaths would be prevented. Long-term investments would have even greater effects.

We know what works to effectively reduce tobacco use, and if we were to fully invest in and implement these proven strategies, we could significantly reduce the staggering toll that tobacco takes on our families and in our communities. We could accelerate the declines in cardiovascular mortality, reduce chronic obstructive pulmonary disease, and make lung cancer a rare disease. With sustained implementation of state tobacco control programs and policies, the *Healthy People 2020* objective of reducing adult smoking prevalence to 12% or less by 2020 could be attainable.

Introduction

Burden of Tobacco Use

Tobacco use is the single most preventable cause of disease and death in the United States.[1] The health consequences of tobacco use include heart disease, multiple types of cancer, pulmonary disease, adverse reproductive effects, and the exacerbation of chronic health conditions.[1] Nearly one-half million Americans still die prematurely from tobacco use each year, and economic costs attributable to smoking and exposure to secondhand smoke now approach $300 billion annually.[2] Despite these known health and financial burdens, approximately one in four American adults currently use some form of tobacco, with one in five smoking cigarettes.[3,4]

This public health problem is compounded by the fact that the harmful effects of tobacco use do not end with the user. Although substantial progress has been made in the adoption of comprehensive smokefree policies that prohibit smoking in all indoor areas of workplaces and public places, millions of Americans not protected by such policies remain susceptible to involuntary secondhand smoke exposure in these areas, as well as private settings such as multiunit housing.[5,6] There is no risk-free level of secondhand smoke, and exposure can cause premature death and disease in nonsmoking adults and children.[7,8]

Nearly 90% of adult smokers begin smoking by the time they are 18 years of age.[9] Although the prevalence of cigarette smoking among youth decreased significantly from the late 1990s to 2003, the rate of decline has slowed in recent years.[10] In 2012, approximately 6.7% of middle school students and 23.3% of high school students reported using a tobacco product within the past 30 days.[11] Several factors may have contributed to this lack of continued decline, including smaller annual increases in the retail price of cigarettes, decreased exposure among youth to effective mass media tobacco control campaigns, and less funding for comprehensive statewide tobacco control programs.[12]

Additionally, actions by the tobacco industry, including substantial increases in expenditures on advertising and promotion at the point of sale, may also have played a role, especially given the industry's history of deceptive advertising. In the 2006 final opinion in United States v. Philip Morris, U.S. District Judge Gladys Kessler concluded that the major tobacco companies are adjudicated racketeers that had "mounted a coordinated, well-financed, sophisticated public relations campaign to attack and distort the scientific evidence demonstrating the relationship between smoking and disease."[13]

Goals of Comprehensive Tobacco Control Programs

In 2007, the Institute of Medicine (IOM) released the report, *Ending the Tobacco Problem: A Blueprint for the Nation,* which outlined a two-pronged strategy for eliminating the burden of tobacco use in the United States.[14] This strategy included: 1) strengthening and fully implementing traditional tobacco control measures; and 2) changing the regulatory landscape to permit policy innovations. The IOM Committee specifically concluded that there was compelling evidence that comprehensive state tobacco programs can achieve substantial reductions in tobacco use.[14]

The mission of comprehensive tobacco control programs is to reduce disease, disability, and death related to tobacco use. A comprehensive approach—one that optimizes synergy from applying a mix of educational, clinical, regulatory, economic, and social strategies—is the guiding principle for eliminating the health and economic burden of tobacco use.[15,16]

Goals for Comprehensive Tobacco Control Programs

- Prevent initiation among youth and young adults.
- Promote quitting among adults and youth.
- Eliminate exposure to secondhand smoke.
- Identify and eliminate tobacco-related disparities among population groups.

Impact of Comprehensive Tobacco Control Programs

States that have made larger investments in comprehensive tobacco control programs have seen larger declines in cigarettes sales than the United States as a whole, and the prevalence of smoking among adults and youth has declined faster as spending for tobacco control programs has increased.[17-19] For example, during 1998–2003, a comprehensive prevention program in Florida anchored by an aggressive youth-oriented health communications campaign reduced the prevalence of smoking among middle and high school students by 50% and 35%, respectively.[20] Similarly, during 2001–2010, the New York State Tobacco Control Program reported declines in the prevalence of smoking among adults and youth in the state that outpaced declines nationally. As a result, smoking-attributable personal health care expenditures in New York in 2010 were $4.1 billion less than they would have been had the prevalence of smoking remained at 2001 levels.[21]

In addition to the beneficial impact of larger investments in comprehensive tobacco control programs on smoking rates, research also shows that the longer states invest in such programs, the greater and quicker the impact.[16] For example, in California, the nation's first and longest-running comprehensive state tobacco control program, the prevalence of smoking among adults declined from 22.7% in 1988 to 11.9% in 2010.[22] Decreases in lung cancer incidence and the correlation between lung cancer incidence and quit ratios also provide compelling evidence of the value of sustained tobacco control efforts. Since 1998, lung cancer incidence in California has been declining four times faster than in the rest of the United States.[23]

National Initiatives to Support Comprehensive Tobacco Control Programs

A comprehensive approach to tobacco prevention and control requires coordination and collaboration across the federal government, across the nation, and within each state. The federal government has undertaken a number of important activities that provide a foundation for state action. For example, in 1999, the National Tobacco Control Program (NTCP) was launched, combining initiatives from the National Cancer Institute (NCI) and the Centers for Disease Control and Prevention (CDC) into one coordinated national program that CDC funds and manages.[24] CDC funding is designed to support and leverage state funding for evidence-based interventions and to help states evaluate their program efforts. NTCP provides technical assistance and limited funding to all 50 states, the District of Columbia, and seven territories, as well as Tribal Support Centers and National Networks of specific populations.

Similarly, The National Network of Tobacco Cessation Quitlines was developed through a partnership among CDC, the NCI Cancer Information Service, the North American Quitline Consortium, and the states.[25] This system provides callers from across the nation with a single, toll-free access point (1-800-QUIT NOW) that automatically routes them to their state's telephone-based cessation services.

In addition to these activities, several major advances were made in recent years through the enactment of national tobacco control legislation. Specifically, the 2009 Family Smoking Prevention and Tobacco Control Act gives the Food and Drug Administration authority to regulate the manufacture, distribution, and marketing of tobacco products.[26] In addition, the Patient Protection and Affordable Care Act, as amended by the Health Care and Education Reconciliation Act and referred to collectively as the Affordable Care Act, provides expanded coverage for recommended clinical preventive services, including evidence-based smoking-cessation treatments, for many persons in the United States.[27] Finally, the Children's Health Insurance Program Reauthorization Act of 2009 raised the federal tax rate for cigarettes from $0.39 to $1.01 per pack.[28] Increasing the price of tobacco products is the single most effective way to prevent initiation among nonsmokers and to reduce consumption.[15,29]

Scientific data about the extent of tobacco use, its impact, and effective interventions to reduce its use have been generated and disseminated by several federal agencies, including CDC, the National Institutes of Health (NIH), the Substance Abuse and Mental Health Services Administration (SAMHSA), and the Agency for Healthcare Research and Quality. The federal government has also supported several national and state tobacco use surveys among adults and youth through the CDC (e.g. Behavioral Risk Factor Surveillance System, National

Health Interview Survey, Youth Risk Behavior Surveillance System, national and state Adult Tobacco Surveys, national and state Youth Tobacco Surveys), NIH (e.g. Tobacco Use Supplement to the Current Population Survey and Monitoring the Future), and SAMHSA (e.g. National Survey on Drug Use and Health). These surveys provide complementary data from various populations that are critical for surveillance and evaluation.

National partner organizations and many academic and research partners also play a critical role in tobacco prevention and control efforts. For example:

- The American Cancer Society, American Heart Association, and American Lung Association provide strong national, state, and local advocacy leadership on tobacco control policy issues as well as community support

- The American Legacy Foundation's truth® campaign reinforces state-based youth prevention efforts and has been independently associated with substantial declines in the prevalence of smoking among youth[30]

- The Americans for Nonsmokers' Rights Foundation provides technical assistance to states and localities as they engage in the process of implementing smokefree policies

- The Association of State and Territorial Health Officials, the National Association of County and City Health Officials, and the National Association of Local Boards of Health provide state and local health officials with support in developing and maintaining tobacco control policies and programs

- The Campaign for Tobacco-Free Kids provides legal, media, and research support to assist in promoting and implementing tobacco control policies

- The Robert Wood Johnson Foundation has supported research to document the effectiveness of policies and programs and also helps build tobacco control infrastructure

- The Tobacco Control Legal Consortium, a network of legal programs supporting tobacco control policy change, works to assist communities and increase legal resources available for tobacco control

- The Tobacco Technical Assistance Consortium supports the effectiveness of tobacco control programs by providing technical assistance to state and local programs, partners, and coalitions

Although a number of critical efforts to curb tobacco use occur at the national level, state and local community action is essential to ensure the success of tobacco control interventions. Most funding for tobacco control interventions comes from the states.[31] Furthermore, it is the policies, partnerships, and intervention activities that occur at the state and local levels that ultimately lead to social norm and behavior change. In acknowledging the essential and unique roles that states and communities play in tobacco control efforts, this report provides technical information and evidence-based benchmarks to assist states in designing comprehensive programs. Communities, in turn, support comprehensive programs by implementing evidence-based initiatives at the local level. For example, although the centralized quitline number and structure of the National Network of Tobacco Cessation Quitlines were established through partnerships at the national level, states still provide the foundation for this system by maintaining their quitline services and promoting their use through broadcast media. Communities can further promote this service through local channels, such as hospitals, health care systems, newspapers, and community organizations.

Implementing Best Practices for Comprehensive Tobacco Control Programs

Evidence-based, statewide tobacco control programs that are comprehensive, sustained, and accountable have been shown to reduce smoking rates as well as tobacco-related diseases and deaths. A comprehensive statewide tobacco control program is a coordinated effort to:

- Establish smokefree policies and social norms

- Promote cessation and assist tobacco users to quit

- Prevent initiation of tobacco use

CDC's *Best Practices for Comprehensive Tobacco Control Programs—2014* is an evidence-based guide to help states plan and establish comprehensive tobacco control programs. CDC has prepared this report to help states organize their tobacco control program efforts into an integrated and effective structure that uses and maximizes interventions proven to be effective and to operate at the scale that would be required to reach the *Healthy People 2020* objective of reducing smoking to 12% or less by the year 2020.

In 1999, CDC first published *Best Practices for Comprehensive Tobacco Control Programs*. That report outlined the elements of an evidence-based state tobacco control program and provided a recommended state funding range to substantially reduce tobacco-related disease, disability, and death.[32] *Best Practices—1999* recommended that states invest a combined $1.6 to $4.2 billion annually in such programs. Subsequently, the recommendation was updated to $3.7 billion annually in 2007.[16]

After the 1999 report was published, overall funding for state tobacco control programs more than doubled, and states restructured their tobacco control programs to align with CDC's goals and programmatic recommendations.[16] To date, all 50 states and the District of Columbia have state tobacco control programs that are funded through various revenue streams, including tobacco industry settlement payments, cigarette excise tax revenues, state general funds, the federal government, and nonprofit organizations.[31]

However, in 2011, only two states funded tobacco control programs at CDC-recommended levels, whereas 27 states funded at less than 25% of these levels.[4] Many state programs have experienced and are facing substantial state government cuts to tobacco control funding, resulting in the near-elimination of tobacco control programs in those states.[31] In 2010, states appropriated only 2.4% of their state tobacco revenues for tobacco control. Reaching the *Best Practices—2007* funding goal would have required an additional 13.0% of tobacco revenues, or $3.1 billion of the $24 billion collected across all states.[31]

Investing in comprehensive tobacco control programs and implementing evidence-based interventions have been shown to reduce youth initiation, tobacco-related disease and death, and tobacco-related health care costs and lost productivity.[14,16,32] These interventions include:

- Increasing the price of tobacco products
- Enacting comprehensive smokefree policies
- Funding hard hitting mass-media campaigns
- Making cessation services fully accessible to tobacco users

Best Practices for Comprehensive Tobacco Control Programs—2014 updates the guidance provided in 2007, reflecting additional state experiences in implementing comprehensive tobacco control programs, new scientific literature, and changes in state populations, inflation, and the national tobacco control landscape.

This report draws upon best practices determined by evidence-based analysis of state tobacco control programs and published evidence of effective tobacco control strategies. On the basis of this analysis, experience, and evidence, CDC recommends that states establish and sustain comprehensive tobacco control programs that contain the following overarching components.

Overarching Components of Comprehensive Tobacco Control Programs

- State and community interventions.
- Mass-reach health communication interventions.
- Cessation interventions.
- Surveillance and evaluation.
- Infrastructure, administration, and management.

This report describes an integrated budget structure for implementing interventions proven to be effective, and the *minimum* and *recommended* state investment that would be required to reduce, and ultimately eliminate, tobacco use in each state. Information for each of these components includes:

- Justification for the program intervention
- Considerations for achieving equity to reduce tobacco-related disparities
- Budget recommendations for successful implementation
- References to assist with implementation

As with the funding guidance published in 2007, annual funding levels can vary within the lower and upper estimate provided for each state.[16] The levels of annual investment for state and community interventions factor in multiple state-specific variables, such as the proportion of individuals within the state living at or below 200% of the poverty level, the proportion of the population that is a racial/ethnic minority, average wage rates for implementing public health programs, geographic size, and the state's infrastructure as reflected by the number of local governmental health units.

The 2014 funding formulas are provided in Appendix A of this report. On the basis of these different factors, the annual investment needed to implement the recommended program components of a comprehensive tobacco control program has been estimated to range from $7.41 to $10.53 per capita for all 50 states and the District of Columbia combined.

The *minimum* and *recommended* funding levels presented in this report reflect the annual investment that each state can make in order to fully fund and sustain a comprehensive tobacco control program. The *minimum* funding level represents the lowest annual investment for attaining a comprehensive tobacco control program. The *recommended* funding level represents the annual level of investment for ensuring a fully funded and sustained comprehensive tobacco control program with resources sufficient to most effectively reduce tobacco use. These funding investment recommendations reflect, in aggregate, a nationally realistic level of investment. States that invest resources above the *recommended* level will accelerate their progress in eliminating tobacco use and reducing tobacco-related morbidity and mortality, and associated costs.

It is important to note that additional investments are also required at the societal level in order to most effectively reduce tobacco use. For example, the enactment of the Affordable Care Act has presented significant new opportunities to institutionalize tobacco use screening and interventions and to increase access to evidence-based cessation treatments through expanded insurance coverage. These costs are important to consider for the purposes of addressing tobacco use but are not necessarily within the purview of state tobacco control program funding parameters. In fact, the new opportunities realized through the Affordable Care Act, along with other factors, contributed to a decline in the recommended state funding levels for cessation interventions in *Best Practices for Comprehensive Tobacco Control Programs—2014*.

Although each state's analysis of their priorities can shape decisions about funding allocations for each recommended program component, it remains clear that more substantial investments in comprehensive state tobacco controls programs lead to quicker and greater declines in smoking rates and in smoking-related disease and death.[17–19]

This report provides evidence to support each of the five components of a comprehensive tobacco control program. While acknowledging the importance of the individual program components, it is critical to recognize why these individual components must work together to produce the synergistic effects of a comprehensive program. A comprehensive approach, with the combination and coordination of all five program components, has shown to be most effective at preventing tobacco use initiation and promoting cessation.[33–35]

Each day in the Unites States, the tobacco industry spends nearly $23 million to advertise and promote cigarettes.[36] During the same period, more than 3,200 youth younger than 18 years of age smoke their first cigarette and another 2,100 youth and young adults who are occasional smokers progress to become daily smokers.[2] However, the tobacco use epidemic can be stopped by implementing the interventions that we know work. Full implementation of comprehensive tobacco control policies and evidence-based interventions at CDC-recommended funding levels would result in a substantial reduction in tobacco-related morbidity and mortality and billions of dollars in savings from averted medical costs and lost productivity in the United States.[2,16]

References

1. U.S. Department of Health and Human Services. *The Health Consequences of Smoking: A Report of the Surgeon General.* Atlanta: U.S. Department of Health and Human Services, Centers for Disease Control and Prevention, National Center for Chronic Disease Prevention and Health Promotion, Office on Smoking and Health, 2004.

2. U.S. Department of Health and Human Services. *The Health Consequences of Smoking – 50 Years of Progress: A Report of the Surgeon General.* Atlanta, GA: U.S. Department of Health and Human Services, Centers for Disease Control and Prevention, Coordinating Center for Health Promotion, National Center for Chronic Disease Prevention and Health Promotion, Office on Smoking and Health, 2014.

3. King BA, Dube SR, Tynan MA. Current tobacco use among adults in the United States: findings from the national Adult Tobacco Survey. *American Journal of Public Health* 2012;102(11):e93–e100.

4. Centers for Disease Control and Prevention. Current cigarette smoking among adults — United States, 2011. *Morbidity and Mortality Weekly Report* 2012;61(44):889–94.

5. Centers for Disease Control and Prevention. Vital signs: nonsmokers' exposure to secondhand smoke — United States, 1999–2008. *Morbidity and Mortality Weekly Report* 2010;59(35):1141–6.

6. Centers for Disease Control and Prevention. State smoke-free laws for worksites, restaurants, and bars — United States, 2000–2010. *Morbidity and Mortality Weekly Report* 2011;60(15):472–5.

7. U.S. Department of Health and Human Services. *The Health Consequences of Involuntary Exposure to Tobacco Smoke: A Report of the Surgeon General.* Atlanta: U.S. Department of Health and Human Services, Centers for Disease Control and Prevention, Coordinating Center for Health Promotion, National Center for Chronic Disease Prevention and Health Promotion, Office on Smoking and Health, 2006.

8. U.S. Department of Health and Human Services. *How Tobacco Smoke Causes Disease: The Biology and Behavioral Basis for Smoking-Attributable Disease: A Report of the Surgeon General.* Atlanta: U.S. Department of Health and Human Services, Centers for Disease Control and Prevention, National Center for Chronic Disease Prevention and Health Promotion, Office on Smoking and Health, 2010.

9. U.S. Department of Health and Human Services. *Preventing Tobacco Use Among Youth and Young Adults.* Atlanta: U.S. Department of Health and Human Services, Centers for Disease Control and Prevention, National Center for Chronic Disease Prevention and Health Promotion, Office on Smoking and Health, 2012.

10. Centers for Disease Control and Prevention. Cigarette use among high school students — United States, 1991–2009. *Morbidity and Mortality Weekly Report* 2010;59(26):797–801.

11. Centers for Disease Control and Prevention. Tobacco product use among middle and high school students — United States, 2011 and 2012. *Morbidity and Mortality Weekly Report* 2013;62(45):893–7.

12. Centers for Disease Control and Prevention. Cigarette use among high school students — United States, 1991–2005. *Morbidity and Mortality Weekly Report* 2006;55(26):724–6.

13. *U.S. v. Philip Morris*, 449 F.Supp.2d 1. D.D.C. 2006.

14. Institute of Medicine. *Ending the Tobacco Problem: A Blueprint for the Nation.* Washington: National Academies Press, 2007.

15. U.S. Department of Health and Human Services. *Reducing Tobacco Use. A Report of the Surgeon General.* Atlanta: U.S. Department of Health and Human Services, Centers for Disease Control and Prevention, National Center for Chronic Disease Prevention and Health Promotion, Office on Smoking and Health, 2000.

16. Centers for Disease Control and Prevention. *Best Practices for Comprehensive Tobacco Control Programs — October 2007.* Atlanta: U.S. Department of Health and Human Services, Centers for Disease Control and Prevention, National Center for Chronic Disease Prevention and Health Promotion, Office on Smoking and Health, 2007.

17. Farrelly MC, Pechacek TF, Chaloupka FJ. The impact of tobacco control program expenditures on aggregate cigarette sales: 1981–2000. *Journal of Health Economics* 2003;22(5):843–59.

18. Tauras JA, Chaloupka FJ, Farrelly MC, Giovino GA, Wakefield M, Johnston LD, O'Malley PM, Kloska DD, Pechacek TF. State tobacco control spending and youth smoking. *American Journal of Public Health* 2005;954(2):338–44.

19. Farrelly MC, Pechacek TF, Thomas KY, Nelson D. The impact of tobacco control programs on adult smoking. *American Journal of Public Health* 2008;89(2):304–9.

20. Bauer UE, Johnson TM, Hopkins RS, Brooks RG. Changes in youth cigarette use and intentions following implementation of a tobacco control program. *JAMA: the Journal of the American Medical Association* 2000;284(6):723–8.

21. RTI International. *2011 Independent Evaluation Report of the New York Tobacco Control Program.* Albany, NY: New York State Department of Health, 2011.

22. California Department of Public Health. Smoking prevalence among California adults, 1984–2010; <http://www.cdph.ca.gov/Pages/NR11-031SmokingChart.aspx>; accessed: December 2, 2013.

23. Centers for Disease Control and Prevention. State-specific trends in lung cancer incidence and smoking — United States, 1999–2008. *Morbidity and Mortality Weekly Report* 2011;60(36):1243–7.

24. Centers for Disease Control and Prevention. National Tobacco Control Program; <http://www.cdc.gov/tobacco/tobacco_control_programs/ntcp/>; accessed: December 2, 2013.

25. U.S. Department of Health and Human Services. HHS Announces National Smoking Cessation Quitline Network; <http://archive.hhs.gov/news/press/2004pres/20040203.html>; accessed: December 2, 2013.

26. *Family Smoking Prevention and Tobacco Control and Federal Retirement Reform.* Public Law 111-31, *U.S. Statutes at Large* 123 (2009):1776; <http://www.gpo.gov/fdsys/pkg/PLAW-111publ31/pdf/PLAW-111publ31.pdf >; accessed: December 2, 2013.

27. *Patient Protection and Affordable Care Act.* Public Law 111-148, *U.S. Statutes at Large* 124 (2010):119; <http://www.gpo.gov/fdsys/pkg/PLAW-111publ148/pdf/PLAW-111publ148.pdf >; accessed: December 2, 2013.

28. *Children's Health Insurance Program Reauthorization Act of 2009.* Public Law 111-3, U.S. Statutes at Large 123 (2009):8; <http://www.gpo.gov/fdsys/pkg/PLAW-111publ3/pdf/PLAW-111publ3.pdf>; accessed: December 2, 2013.

29. Centers for Disease Control and Prevention. Federal and state cigarette excise taxes — United States, 1995–2009. *Morbidity and Mortality Weekly Report* 2009;58(19):524–7.

30. Farrelly MC, Davis KC, Haviland L, Messeri P, Healton CG. Evidence of a dose-response relationship between "truth" antismoking ads and youth smoking prevalence. *American Journal of Public Health* 2005;95(3):425–31.

31. Centers for Disease Control and Prevention. State tobacco revenues compared with tobacco control appropriations — United States, 1998–2010. *Morbidity and Mortality Weekly Report* 2012;61(20):370–4.

32. Centers for Disease Control and Prevention. *Best Practices for Comprehensive Tobacco Control Programs — August 1999.* Atlanta: U.S. Department of Health and Human Services, Centers for Disease Control and Prevention, National Center for Chronic Disease Prevention and Health Promotion, Office on Smoking and Health, 1999.

33. Zaza S, Briss PA, Harris KW, editors. *The Guide to Community Preventive Services: What Works to Promote Health?* New York: Oxford University Press, 2005.

34. Eriksen, M. Lessons learned from public health efforts and their relevance to preventing childhood obesity. In: Koplan JP, Liverman CT, Kraak VA, editors. *Preventing Childhood Obesity: Health in the Balance.* Washington: National Academy of Sciences; 2005:343–75.

35. National Cancer Institute. *Greater Than the Sum: Systems Thinking in Tobacco Control. Tobacco Control* Monograph No. 18. Bethesda (MD): U.S. Department of Health and Human Services, Public Health Service, National Institutes of Health, National Cancer Institute, 2007. NIH Publication No. 06-6085.

36. Federal Trade Commission. Federal Trade Commission Cigarette Report for 2011; <http://www.ftc.gov/os/2013/05/130521cigarettereport.pdf>; accessed: December 2, 2013.

Section A
Components of a Comprehensive Tobacco Control Program

I. State and Community Interventions

Justification

The history of successful public health practice has demonstrated that the active and coordinated involvement of a wide range of societal and community resources must be the foundation of sustained solutions to pervasive problems like tobacco use.[1-8] In a review of evidence of population-wide tobacco prevention and control efforts, the Task Force on Community Preventive Services confirmed the importance of coordinated and combined intervention efforts.[9] The strongest evidence demonstrating the effectiveness of many of the population-wide approaches that are most highly recommended by the Task Force on Community Preventive Services comes from studies in which specific strategies for smoking cessation, preventing tobacco use initiation, and eliminating exposure to secondhand smoke are combined with mass-media campaigns and efforts to mobilize communities and to integrate these strategies into synergistic and multicomponent efforts.[9]

Additionally, research has demonstrated the importance of community support and involvement at the grassroots level in implementing several of the most highly effective policy interventions, including increasing the unit price of tobacco products and creating smokefree public and private environments.[3,4,6,10-12] Although knowledge is critical, communities must reinforce and support health.[13] Example program and policy recommendations from the Task Force on Community Preventive Services, as well as the *Healthy People 2020* policy goals for the nation, are provided in Appendix B. In addition, recommendations for tobacco-free living from the National Prevention Council are provided in Appendix C.

The policies, partnerships, and intervention activities that occur at the state and community levels will ultimately lead to social norm and behavior change nationwide. State and community coalitions are essential partnerships. For example, they can keep tobacco issues before the public, combat the tobacco industry, enhance community involvement and promote community buy-in and support, educate policy makers, and help to inform policy change.

Social norm change influences behavior indirectly by creating social and legal climates in which harmful products and conduct become less desirable, acceptable, and attainable. The health impact pyramid provides a five-tier framework to improve health through different types of public health interventions, with greater improvements coming from activities focused on policy change that create a context in which the healthy options are easy to attain.[6] This community intervention model has now become a core element of statewide comprehensive tobacco control programs.[3,4,10,14-16]

Since the establishment of the California Tobacco Control Program in 1989, California has achieved an almost 50% decline in the prevalence of smoking among adults, from 22.7% in 1988 to 11.9% in 2010; nearly one million lives saved from a combination of smokers who quit and young people who chose not to start; and improved health outcomes for Californians, with lung cancer declining nearly four times faster than in the rest of the nation.[17] During fiscal years 1989–2008, the California Tobacco Control Program cost $2.4 billion and led to cumulative health care expenditure savings of $134 billion.[18] The program uses a social-norm-change approach to reduce the uptake and continued use of tobacco products. For example, the statewide media campaign frames the message, community-level projects provide education on evidence-based tobacco control policy interventions, and statewide projects build the capacity of community-level projects. The tobacco control program's technical assistance is the engine powering social change across California by playing a key role in the education of evidence-based policy approaches to reduce tobacco use.[19] State comprehensive tobacco control programs nationwide have the tools to match and even exceed California's achievements.

Tobacco control interventions can counter the aggressive and often misleading information spread by tobacco companies, which have been found in federal court to have deliberately deceived the public about the health effects of tobacco.[20] In this context, it is particularly important that comprehensive statewide tobacco control programs coordinate community-level interventions that counter tobacco industry marketing and focus on:

Section A: State and Community Interventions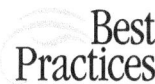

- Preventing initiation among youth and young adults
- Promoting quitting among adults and youth
- Eliminating exposure to secondhand smoke
- Identifying and eliminating tobacco-related disparities among population groups

Reducing tobacco use is particularly challenging because tobacco products are so heavily marketed. In 2011, tobacco companies spent more than $8 billion, or nearly $23 million per day, to market cigarettes in the United States, mostly at the point of sale.[21] In addition to these tobacco advertising and promotion efforts, both adults and youth have been, and continue to be, heavily exposed to images of smoking in the movies, other mass-media, social marketing, and digital and mobile technologies.[22–26] For example, 35% of U.S. youth reported having seen tobacco advertisements on the Internet in 2008.[7] Research has shown that there is a causal relationship between advertising and promotional efforts of the tobacco companies and the initiation and progression of tobacco use among young people;[7] approximately one-third of underage experimentation with smoking can be attributed to tobacco industry advertising and promotion.[7]

As cigarette use declines, new tobacco products, such as noncombustible products, and nicotine delivery products, such as e-cigarettes, are also being introduced and marketed. Approximately one of five current smokers has used e-cigarettes.[27] Additionally, e-cigarette experimentation and recent use doubled among U.S. middle and high school students during 2011–2012, resulting in an estimated 1.78 million students having ever used e-cigarettes as of 2012.[28] Coordinated implementation of a broad range of statewide and community programs and policies is important to ensuring that the continued marketing of cigarettes and other combustible products, as well as the new marketing and sale of emerging non-combustible products, does not prolong the harms caused by smoking. These programs and policies are best implemented along with mass media campaigns to influence societal organizations, systems, and networks that encourage and support individuals to make behavior choices consistent with tobacco-free norms.[3,4,14,29,30]

Community engagement is essential for meaningful change to occur in the way that tobacco products are marketed, sold, and used. The National Association of County and City Health Officials has developed guidelines for comprehensive local tobacco control programs (Appendix D).[31] The CDC-recommended community-based model to produce durable changes in social norms is based on evidence that approaches with the greatest span (economic, regulatory, and comprehensive) and jurisdictional reach (number of people covered) will have the greatest population impact.[3,4,14,29,30]

Interventions to prevent tobacco use initiation and to encourage cessation among youth and young adults can reshape the environment so that it supports tobacco-free norms. Nearly 9 of 10 smokers in the United States start smoking by the time they are 18 years old, and 99% start by the age of 26.[7] Thus, intervening during adolescence and young adulthood is critical.[32] Research has shown that increasing the unit price of tobacco products, comprehensive smokefree air laws, and state tobacco control programs are effective strategies for curbing youth and adult smoking.[32] Community programs and school and college policies and interventions should be part of a comprehensive effort—coordinated and implemented in conjunction with efforts to create tobacco-free social norms, including increasing the unit price of tobacco products, sustaining anti-tobacco media campaigns, and making environments smokefree.[7,9,22,33]

Recommendations for Preventing Tobacco Use Among Youth[9,34]

- Increase the unit price of tobacco products.
- Conduct mass-media education campaigns in combination with other community interventions.
- Mobilize the community to restrict minors' access to tobacco products in combination with additional interventions (stronger local laws directed at retailers, active enforcement of retailer sales laws, and retailer education with reinforcement).

Most states fund community and statewide organizations to develop and maintain an infrastructure and to implement population-wide and specific programs. To achieve lasting changes, community and statewide organizations require funding to hire diverse staff, provide operating expenses, purchase or develop education materials and resources, conduct education and training programs, carry out communication and media advocacy campaigns, and recruit and maintain local partnerships.[31]

Statewide Programs

Statewide programs can deliver statewide programming such as mass media campaigns and enforcement efforts, and provide leadership and coordination of efforts related to state policies, laws, and regulations. Statewide programs also can provide the skills, resources, and information needed for coordinated and strategic implementation of effective community programs. For example, training local community coalitions about the legal and technical aspects of comprehensive smokefree policies and enforcement can be provided most efficiently through statewide partners who have experience in administering these services. In states where comprehensive smokefree policies have already been implemented, efforts to promote smokefree private environments, such as multiunit housing, may be considered. Direct funding provided to statewide organizations can be used to mobilize their organizational assets to strengthen statewide initiatives and community resources.

For example, the New York Tobacco Control Program runs statewide media campaigns, develops and executes policy and regulatory initiatives, implements enforcement efforts, and funds organizations across the state to work in five modalities: community partnerships for tobacco control, youth action programs, school policy programs, cessation centers, and colleges for change programs. Community programs are structured in such a way that every county falls within the coverage area of a community partnership, a cessation center, and a school policy program. All community programs are charged with bringing about environmental change in multiple settings, including worksites, schools, licensed tobacco retailers, multiunit housing, and public spaces such as parks and beaches. These community actions complement and reinforce similar statewide action through three types of activities: use of paid and earned media to raise awareness and educate the community and key community members about the tobacco epidemic; education of government policy makers about the tobacco epidemic to build support for tobacco control policies; and education of organizational decision makers, including tobacco retailers, health care organizations, school boards, and community organizations, for policy changes and resolutions.[35]

It is important to note that careful attention must be paid to ensuring that public funds are appropriately used. Tracking and reporting on funding sources by activity is integral to ensure that public funds are not used for prohibited activities.

CDC's National Center for Chronic Disease Prevention and Health Promotion has developed four domains that can provide a framework for state tobacco prevention and control programs to collaborate with other state and community programs to address diseases for which tobacco is a major cause, including multiple cancers, heart disease and stroke, and chronic lung and respiratory diseases (See Figure 1).[36]

Figure 1. Key domains for transforming the nation's health and providing individuals with equitable opportunities to take charge of their health.

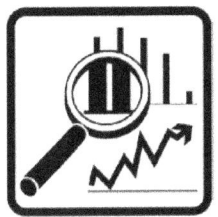

Domain 1
Epidemiology and surveillance to gather, analyze, and disseminate data and information and conduct evaluation to inform, prioritize, deliver, and monitor programs and population health.

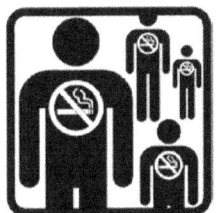

Domain 2
Environmental approaches that promote health and support and reinforce healthful behaviors statewide and in communities.

Domain 3
Health system interventions to improve the effective delivery and use of clinical and other preventive services in order to prevent disease, detect diseases early, and reduce or eliminate risk factors and mitigate or manage complications.

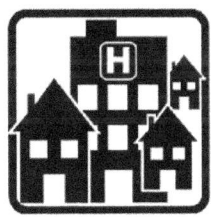

Domain 4
Strategies to improve community-clinical linkages ensuring that communities support and clinics refer patients to programs that improve management of chronic conditions.

Addressing evidence-based tobacco control strategies in the broader context of tobacco-related diseases is beneficial for four reasons:

- It is critical that interventions are implemented to alleviate the existing burden of tobacco-related disease.
- The incorporation of tobacco prevention and cessation messages into broader public health activities ensures wider dissemination of tobacco control strategies.
- Tobacco use in conjunction with other diseases and risk factors, such as sedentary lifestyle, poor diet, and diabetes, poses a greater combined risk and poorer prognosis for many chronic diseases than the sum of each individual degree of risk.
- Educating the public about the broader context of tobacco-related diseases helps mobilize public support and action for tobacco control.

Each state's financial, social, and demographic characteristics have a significant role in tobacco prevention and control efforts. Examples are provided in the following box.

Examples of Statewide Efforts for Tobacco Prevention and Control

- Supporting and/or facilitating tobacco prevention and control partnership and coalition development, as well as links to other related partnerships and coalitions (e.g., cancer control, cardiovascular disease, diabetes, asthma).

- Establishing a strategic plan for comprehensive tobacco control with appropriate partners at the state and community levels.

- Educating state leaders, decision-makers, and the public about the burden of tobacco use and evidence-based policy and other strategies to reduce this burden.

- Engaging stakeholders and partners on approaches, such as message development and messengers, to reach populations with the greatest disparities in tobacco use.

- Collecting, disseminating, and analyzing state and community-specific data; developing and implementing culturally appropriate interventions with appropriate multicultural involvement; and making program adjustments as indicated.

- Sponsoring community, regional, and statewide trainings, conferences, and technical assistance on best practices for effective tobacco use prevention and cessation programs.

- Monitoring pro-tobacco influences to facilitate public discussion and debate among partners, decision makers, and other stakeholders at the state and community level.

- Supporting community-level innovations in tobacco control that may enhance the public health impact of current state-level policies and disseminating successful interventions across communities.

Community Programs

A "community" encompasses a diverse set of entities that reach across multiple sectors, including voluntary health agencies; civic, social, and recreational organizations; businesses and business associations; city and county governments; public health organizations; labor groups; health care systems and providers; health care professionals' societies; schools and universities; faith organizations; and organizations for racial and ethnic minority groups.[1–5,8,10]

To counter aggressive pro-tobacco influences, communities are encouraged to change the knowledge, attitudes, and practices of tobacco users and nonusers and also engage in strategies to address the manner in which tobacco is promoted, the time, manner, and place in which tobacco is sold, and how and where tobacco is used.[4,5,7]

State and local governments play an integral role in achieving the goals of the Family Smoking Prevention and Tobacco Control Act (FSPTCA), which granted the Food and Drug Administration (FDA) the authority to regulate tobacco products.[37] The FSPTCA permits states and local governments to impose specific bans or restrictions on the time, place, and manner—but not the content—of cigarette advertisements. States may adopt or continue to enforce requirements pertaining to tobacco products that are in addition to, or more stringent than, many requirements of the law. However, although the law preserves a substantial amount of the states' authority to regulate tobacco products, some state and local requirements are preempted.[37]

Effective community programs involve and influence people in their daily environment.[1,3–5,8,38] Therefore, community engagement and mobilization are essential to programs addressing tobacco control.[39,40] Implementing strategies that can impact societal organizations, systems, and networks necessitates the involvement of community partners.[1,2,4,7] Decreasing disparities in tobacco use occurs largely through engagement in evidence-based community interventions.

Examples of State Program Involvement in Community-Level Interventions

- Providing funding to community-based organizations in order to strengthen the capacity of these groups to positively inform social norms regarding tobacco use and to build relationships among multiple sectors of the community, such as housing, education, business, planning, and transport.

- Empowering local agencies to build community coalitions and partnerships that facilitate collaboration among programs in local governments, voluntary and civic organizations, and diverse community-based organizations.

- Collaborating with partners and other programs to implement evidence-based interventions and build and sustain capacity through technical assistance and training.

- Supporting community strategies or efforts to educate the public and media, not only about the health effects of tobacco use and exposure to secondhand smoke, but also about available cessation services.

- Promoting public discussion among partners, decision makers, and other stakeholders about tobacco-related health issues and pro-tobacco influences.

- Establishing a community strategic plan of action that is consistent with the statewide strategic plan.

- Ensuring that funding formulas for the local public health infrastructure provide grantees (e.g., local and county health departments, tribal organizations, nonprofit organizations) operating expenses commensurate with tobacco control program and evaluation efforts.

- Ensuring that community grantees measure and evaluate social norm change outcomes (e.g., policy adoption, increased compliance) resulting from their interventions.

- Ensuring that partners receiving funding for tobacco control from various entities work collaboratively.

Achieving Equity to Eliminate Tobacco-Related Disparities

Reducing tobacco-related disparities is a critical component of a comprehensive tobacco control program.[10,41] Tobacco-related disparities are differences that exist among population groups with regard to key tobacco-related indicators, including patterns, prevention, and treatment of tobacco use; the risk, incidence, morbidity, mortality, and burden of tobacco-related illness; and capacity, infrastructure, and access to resources; and second-hand smoke exposure.[42]

Identifying and eliminating tobacco-related disparities among population groups is one of the four goals for comprehensive state tobacco control programs. To ultimately eliminate tobacco-related disparities, tobacco control programs and policies must be implemented in a way that achieves equitable benefits for all.

Activities focused on achieving equity and eliminating tobacco-related disparities can help accelerate the decline in the prevalence of tobacco use and access to effective cessation treatments, thus alleviating the disproportionate health and economic burden experienced by some population subgroups.[10] Tobacco-related disparities can affect population subgroups on the basis of certain factors, including but not limited to:[43,44]

- Age
- Disability/limitation
- Educational attainment
- Geographic location (e.g., rural/urban)
- Income
- Mental health status
- Occupation
- Race/ethnicity
- Sex
- Sexual orientation and gender identity
- Substance abuse conditions
- Veteran and military status

It is important to use surveillance systems and other data collection systems to measure these types of characteristics within states and communities to help identify populations with tobacco-related disparities,[45] and to engage members of affected communities in reducing and preventing tobacco use.

Activities to Support Equity Achievement and Eliminate Tobacco-Related Disparities

- Conduct surveillance to identify populations disproportionately affected by tobacco use.
- Partner with population groups and community-based organizations that serve these populations experiencing tobacco-related disparities.
- Ensure that health equity is an integral part of state and community tobacco control strategic plans.
- Mitigate barriers to effective implementation of tobacco control interventions, such as enhancing access to cessation services for low-income or other communities.
- Fund organizations that can effectively reach, educate, and involve populations experiencing tobacco-related disparities.
- Provide culturally competent technical assistance and training to grantees and partners.

In order to adequately identify and effectively eliminate tobacco-related disparities, state tobacco control programs must implement a number of tobacco prevention and control strategies, including establishing infrastructure and building capacity.[42] These strategies are useful for guiding the development of policies and practices that reflect the principles of inclusion, cultural competency, and equity. Reaching the national goal of eliminating health disparities related to tobacco use will also require enhanced collection and use of standardized data to correctly identify disparities in tobacco-related outcomes, including awareness and use of tobacco products, health outcomes, and program effectiveness.[45,46] The use of oversampling, combining multiple years of data, and qualitative methods are often necessary to adequately assess these outcomes among some population groups.[10] In addition, clear leadership, dedicated resources, and a commitment to inclusion are essential to develop and implement a strong strategic plan.[42]

Strategies to Achieve Equity and Eliminate Tobacco-Related Disparities

- Create partnerships to maximize resources and reach of interventions.
- Integrate efforts to eliminate tobacco-related disparities in all chronic disease prevention areas.
- Identify and develop culturally competent materials and interventions.
- Educate partners and key decision makers about tobacco-related disparities.
- Reduce exposure to targeted tobacco industry advertising, promotion, and sponsorship.
- Obtain comprehensive Medicaid coverage for tobacco dependence treatments.
- Evaluate intervention efficacy and refine efforts as appropriate.

This guidance is based upon information and experience derived from state practices, scientific studies, and input from external partners and experts in the field of tobacco control. The guidance highlights the presumed minimum capacity and infrastructure needed by state tobacco control programs to pursue a strategic plan with initiatives that will most effectively achieve equity in tobacco prevention and control through the identification and elimination of tobacco-related disparities.[47]

Ending the Epidemic: A Tobacco Control Strategic Action Plan for the U.S. Department of Health and Human Services, which was published in 2010, called attention to the need to reduce tobacco-related disparities through specific interventions in locations serving high-risk populations, such as subsidized and public housing, substance abuse facilities, mental health facilities, correctional institutions, community health centers, federally qualified health centers, Ryan White clinics, rural health clinics, and critical access hospitals.

Reducing the prevalence of tobacco use requires greater attention to populations carrying a disproportionate burden of use and dependence. One way to reach such groups is through efforts that directly affect those populations, including tobacco-free policies, quitline promotion, and counseling and cessation services.[48] Following are examples from select states that have made such efforts.

In 2006, the Massachusetts Medicaid program expanded its cessation benefit by providing comprehensive coverage of tobacco cessation medications.[49] More than 75,000 (37%) Medicaid subscribers used the benefit in the first two and a half years. The prevalence of smoking among the Medicaid population decreased from 38% to 28% during this period. Use of a comprehensive tobacco cessation benefit that includes pharmacotherapy was associated with a significant decrease in claims for hospitalizations for heart attacks and acute coronary heart disease. Annualized hospitalizations for these cardiovascular conditions among Medicaid smokers who used the benefit declined by almost half. Every dollar spent on the benefit was associated with $3.12 in medical savings for cardiovascular conditions.[49]

In California, the California Smoker's Helpline and the Asian Smokers Quitline provide cessation services and culturally appropriate information in multiple languages for different audiences. These focused tobacco cessation interventions, along with other elements, have led to significant reductions in smoking across ethnic groups in California. For instance, during 1990-2005, smoking rates among Asian men dropped from 20% to less than 15%; among Hispanic men, from 22% to 16%; and among African American men, from 28% to 21%.[50]

Adults with any mental illness have a high prevalence of cigarette smoking.[51] Moreover, sociodemographic variations in the prevalence of current smoking among persons with any mental illness resemble patterns in the overall population, and adult smokers with mental illness are less likely to quit than those smokers without mental illness. Accordingly, enhanced prevention and cessation efforts among persons with mental illness can further reduce smoking-related death and disease. For example, the New York tobacco control program has identified populations with chemical addictions or mental illness for specific intervention. To reach these populations, the state used strategies that included integrating tobacco dependence treatment into treatment protocols for mental illness or chemical dependency, promoting tobacco-free campuses for substance abuse and mental health facilities, and partnering with agencies representing each group.[52]

In 2013, the following national networks jointly designed and sponsored a series of trainings in Texas to introduce specific populations to tobacco control: the National African American Tobacco Prevention Network (NAATPN), the National Latino Tobacco Control Network (NLTCN), and the Asian Pacific Partners for Empowerment, Advocacy and Leadership (APPEAL). Participants with long-term involvement in their communities were identified and recruited to attend these training opportunities. The trainings sought to increase specific population leadership, collaboration, and civic engagement at a grassroots level to address disparities in health that result from tobacco use and secondhand smoke exposure. The trainings addressed the importance of: building organizational capacity by connecting participants with local coalitions, including Community Transformation Grantees, or building a local coalition; mobilizing communities to address health disparities and implement tobacco control and health promotion policies; facilitating cross cultural collaboration among Latino, African American, and Asian American, Native Hawaiian, and Pacific Islander communities; increasing leadership knowledge and skills on health disparities among community advocates; increasing knowledge of the impact of tobacco use on chronic disease disparities; creating emerging promising practices on engaging priority populations; and developing materials and approaches, such as workers' rights and social justice, that make secondhand smoke exposure relevant to populations with a high burden of exposure.

Budget

Linking state and community interventions creates synergistic effects, greatly increasing the effects of each comprehensive tobacco control component. Effective actions are those that reinforce one another, including: raising community awareness and mobilization efforts; developing health communication interventions; collecting, analyzing, and disseminating data; and providing cessation interventions. Evidence indicates that interventions that promote changes in social norms appear to be the most effective approach for sustained behavior change.[9]

Best Practices dictates allocating funds for establishing and sustaining internal capacity with experienced staff and developing an infrastructure with partner organizations and other programs to oversee and implement evidence-based programs. Most states fund local health departments, boards of health, or health-related nonprofit community organizations representing each county, multicounty region, or major metropolitan areas to develop and maintain local infrastructure and implement jurisdiction-wide and targeted programs. *Best Practices* recommends that funds be awarded directly to tribal health departments and tribal-serving organizations to deliver tobacco control programming to tribes and tribal members, as well as to other organizations that serve specific populations, in order to implement evidence-based programs and activities with that population. Funds may also be distributed to different agencies to ensure compliance with tobacco prevention and control laws. These varied efforts remain integrated through effective communication, coalitions, and networks. It is important that states also take into account the special issues of different communities within their state, such as large variations in population size, differences in the prevalence of smoking among various populations, access to cessation services, and reach of the interventions.

Recommendations for funding state and community interventions are based on the 1999 funding formulas, which were updated in 2007 to include the following major components: statewide programs, community programs to reduce tobacco use, chronic disease programs to reduce the burden of tobacco-related diseases, school programs, and enforcement.[47,53]

The *minimum* and *recommended* funding levels are derived from the 2007 funding formulas and adjusted for population changes and inflation. The specific state-recommended level of investment is based on the relative complexity and cost of doing business in that state. Drawing from the experience of states that have implemented robust state and community interventions, funding levels were determined for each state. The *minimum* and *recommended* levels of investment were based primarily on each state's current smoking prevalence, while also taking into account other factors such as the proportion of individuals within the state living at or below 200% of the poverty level, the proportion of the population that is a racial/ethnic minority, average wage rates for implementing public health programs, geographic size, and the state's infrastructure as reflected by the number of local governmental health units.

For the 2014 update of *Best Practices*, the state and community interventions formula does not specifically include chronic disease programs to reduce the burden of tobacco-related diseases, school programs, and enforcement as major components. However, activities in these three areas may still be undertaken within the framework of state and community interventions. For example, chronic disease prevention and control programs are stakeholders and partners in tobacco control. Using evidence-based interventions and strategies to address state tobacco control priorities, as described in the state chronic disease plan, can support achieving the four National Tobacco Control Program goals. Similarly, there is little evidence of the long-term effectiveness of school-based programs to prevent smoking.[7,54] However, they can be more efficacious when part of a comprehensive, multicomponent approach to tobacco use prevention that includes school policies, community-wide strategies, and mass media. Finally, active enforcement of youth access laws is part of broader community mobilization efforts that combine additional interventions, including stronger retailer laws and retailer education, with reinforcement. The FSPTCA authorizes FDA to contract with states, territories, and tribes for the purposes of conducting compliance check inspections of tobacco retailers. Some states have contracted with local public health organizations to assist with FDA's rigorous enforcement efforts.

For the last 15 years, states have implemented CDC's recommendations, focusing their efforts on proven activities that have the greatest impact, while also expanding the evidence-base of effective tobacco control interventions and building on each other's successes.[7,9,10,33]

References

1. Green LW, Kreuter M. *Health Promotion Planning: An Educational and Ecological Approach.* New York: McGraw-Hill, 2000.

2. Institute of Medicine. *The Future of Public's Health in the 21st Century.* Washington: National Academies Press, 2002.

3. Eriksen, M. Lessons learned from public health efforts and their relevance to preventing childhood obesity. In: Koplan JP, Liverman CT, Kraak VA, editors. *Preventing Childhood Obesity: Health in the Balance.* Washington: National Academy of Sciences, 2005:343–75.

4. National Cancer Institute. *ASSIST: Shaping the Future of Tobacco Prevention and Control. Tobacco Control* Monograph No. 16. Bethesda (MD): U.S. Department of Health and Human Services, Public Health Service, National Institutes of Health, National Cancer Institute, 2005. NIH Publication No. 05-5645.

5. Cummings KM, Sciandra R, Carol J, Burgess S, Tye JB, Flewelling R. Approaches directed to the social environment. In: *Strategies to Control Tobacco Use in the United States: A Blueprint for Public Health in the 1990's.* Tobacco Control Monograph No. 1. Bethesda (MD): U.S. Department of Health and Human Services, Public Health Service, National Institutes of Health, National Cancer Institute, 1991. NIH Publication 92-3316. Pages 203–65.

6. Frieden, TR. A framework for public health action: the health impact pyramid. *American Journal of Public Health* 2010;100(4):590–5.

7. U.S. Department of Health and Human Services. *Preventing Tobacco Use Among Youth and Young Adults: A Report of the Surgeon General.* Atlanta: U.S. Department of Health and Human Services, Centers for Disease Control and Prevention, National Center for Chronic Disease Prevention and Health Promotion, Office on Smoking and Health, 2012.

8. U.S. Department of Health and Human Services. *Principles of Community Engagement: Second Edition.* National Institutes of Health, Centers for Disease Control and Prevention, and Agency for Toxic Substances and Disease Registry, 2011. NIH Publication No. 11-7782.

9. Zaza S, Briss PA, Harris KW, editors. *The Guide to Community Preventive Services: What Works to Promote Health?* New York: Oxford University Press, 2005.

10. U.S. Department of Health and Human Services. *Reducing Tobacco Use: A Report of the Surgeon General.* Atlanta: U.S. Department of Health and Human Services, Centers for Disease Control and Prevention, National Center for Chronic Disease Prevention and Health Promotion, Office on Smoking and Health, 2000.

11. U.S. Department of Health and Human Services. *The Health Consequences of Involuntary Exposure to Tobacco Smoke: A Report of the Surgeon General.* Atlanta: U.S. Department of Health and Human Services, Centers for Disease Control and Prevention, Coordinating Center for Health Promotion, National Center for Chronic Disease Prevention and Health Promotion, Office on Smoking and Health, 2006.

12. National Cancer Institute. *Community-Based Interventions for Smokers: The COMMIT Field Experience.* Tobacco Control Monograph No. 6. Bethesda (MD): U.S. Department of Health and Human Services, Public Health Service, National Institutes of Health, National Cancer Institute, 1995. NIH Publication No. 95-4028.

13. National Prevention Council. *National Prevention Council Action Plan: Implementing the National Prevention Strategy.* Washington: National Prevention Council, 2012.

14. California Department of Health Services. *A Model for Change: The California Experience in Tobacco Control.* Sacramento, CA: California Department of Health Services, 1998.

15. National Cancer Institute. *Evaluating ASSIST: A Blueprint for Understanding State-Level Tobacco Control.* Tobacco Control Monograph No. 17. Bethesda (MD): U.S. Department of Health and Human Services, Public Health Service, National Institutes of Health, National Cancer Institute, 2006. NIH Publication No. 06-6058.

16. Mueller NB, Luke DA, Herbers SH, Montgomery TP. The best practices: use of the guidelines by ten state tobacco control programs. *American Journal of Preventive Medicine* 2006;31:300–6.

17. California Department of Public Health. *State Health Officer's Report on Tobacco Use and Promotion in California.* California Tobacco Control Program, 2012.

18. Lightwood J, Glantz SA. The effect of the California tobacco control program on smoking prevalence, cigarette consumption, and healthcare costs: 1989–2008. *PLoS One* 2013;8(2):e47145

19. Roeseler A, Hagaman T, Kurtz C. The use of training and technical assistance to drive and improve performance of California's Tobacco Control Program. *Health Promotion Practice* 2011;12(6 Suppl2):130S–143S.

20. Frieden, TR. Government's role in protecting health and safety. *New England Journal of Medicine* 2013;368(20):1857–9.

21. Federal Trade Commission. Federal Trade Commission Cigarette Report for 2011; <http://www.ftc.gov/os/2013/05/130521cigaretterepo rt.pdf>; accessed: December 2, 2013.

22. U.S. Department of Health and Human Services. *Preventing Tobacco Use Among Young People: A Report of the Surgeon General.* Atlanta: U.S. Department of Health and Human Services, Public Health Service, Centers for Disease Control and Prevention, National Center for Chronic Disease Prevention and Health Promotion, Office on Smoking and Health, 1994.

23. Charlesworth A, Glantz SA. Tobacco and the movie industry. *Clinics in Occupational and Environmental Medicine* 2006;5(1):73–84.

24. Cummings KM, Morley CP, Horan JK, Leavell NR. Marketing to America's youth: evidence from corporate documents. *Tobacco Control* 2002;11(Suppl 1):i5–i17.

25. Sargent JD, Stoolmiller M, Worth KA, Dal Cin S, Wills TA, Gibbons FX, et al. Exposure to smoking depictions in movies: its association with established adolescent smoking. *Archives of Pediatric Adolescent Medicine* 2007;161(9):849–56.

26. Dube, SR, Arrazola RA, Lee J, Engstrom M, Malarcher A. Pro-tobacco influences and susceptibility to smoking cigarettes among middle and high school students — United States, 2011. *Journal of Adolescent Health* 2013;52(5 Suppl):45S–51S.

27. King BA, Alam S, Promoff G, Arrazola R, Dube SR. Awareness and ever use of electronic cigarettes among U.S. adults, 2010–2011. *Nicotine & Tobacco Research* 2013;15(9):1623–7.

28. Centers for Disease Control and Prevention. Notes from the field: electronic cigarette use among middle and high school students — United States, 2011–2012. *Morbidity and Mortality Weekly Report* 2013;62(35);729–30.

29. California Department of Health Services. *Communities of Excellence in Tobacco Control.* Sacramento, CA: California Department of Health Services, Tobacco Control Section, 2006.

30. Tobacco Technical Assistance Consortium. Communities of Excellence Plus; <http://www.tacenters.emory.edu/documents/communities_excellence_plus.pdf>; accessed: December 2, 2013.

31. National Association of County and City Health Officials. *Program and Funding Guidelines for Comprehensive Local Tobacco Control Programs (2010).* Washington: National Association of County and City Health Officials, 2010.

32. Farrelly MC, Loomis BR, Han B, Gfroerer J, Kuiper N, Couzens GL, Dube S, Caraballo RS. A comprehensive examination of the influences of state tobacco control programs and policies on youth smoking. *American Journal of Public Health* 2013;103(3):549–55.

33. Institute of Medicine. *Ending the Tobacco Problem: A Blueprint for the Nation.* Washington: National Academies Press, 2007.

34. Task Force on Community Preventive Services. Recommendations regarding interventions to reduce tobacco use and exposure to environmental tobacco smoke. *American Journal of Preventive Medicine* 2001;20(2S):10–5.

35. RTI International. *2010 Independent Evaluation Report for the New York Tobacco Control Program.* Albany, NY: New York State Department of Health, 2010.

36. Centers for Disease Control and Prevention. Chronic Disease Prevention and Health Promotion Domains; <http://www.cdc.gov/chronicdisease/pdf/Four-Domains-Nov2012.pdf>; accessed: December 2, 2013.

37. *Family Smoking Prevention and Tobacco Control Act,* Public Law 111-31, *U.S. Statutes at Large* 123 (2009):1776.

38. Minkler M, editor. *Community Organizing and Community Building for Health.* 2nd edition. New Brunswick, NJ: Rutgers University Press, 2005.

39. Ahmed SM, Palermo AG. Community engagement in research: frameworks for education and peer review. *American Journal of Public Health* 2010;100(8):1380–7.

40. Minkler M, Wallerstein N. The growing support for CPBR. In Minkler M, Wallerstein N, editors. *Community-Based Participatory Research for Health: From Process to Outcomes.* 2nd ed. San Francisco: Jossey-Bass, 2008.

Section A: State and Community Interventions

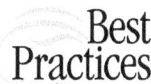

41. U.S. Department of Health and Human Services. *Tobacco Use Among U.S. Racial/Ethnic Minority Groups — African Americans, American Indians and Alaska Natives, Asian Americans and Pacific Islanders, and Hispanics: A Report of the Surgeon General.* Atlanta: U.S. Department of Health and Human Services, Centers for Disease Control and Prevention, Office on Smoking and Health, 1998.

42. Fagan P, King G, Lawrence D, Petrucci SA, Robinson RG, Banks D, et al. Eliminating tobacco-related health disparities: directions for future research. *American Journal of Public Health* 2004;94(2):211–7.

43. Garrett BE, Dube SR, Trosclair A, Caraballo RS, Pechacek TF. Cigarette smoking — United States, 1965–2008. *Morbidity and Mortality Weekly Report* 2011;60(01):109–3.

44. King BA, Dube SR, Tynan MA. Current tobacco use among adults in the United States: findings from the National Adult Tobacco Survey. *American Journal of Public Health* 2012;102(11):e93–e100.

45. Starr G, Rogers T, Schooley M, Porter S, Wiesen E, Jamison N. *Key Outcome Indicators for Evaluating Comprehensive Tobacco Control Programs.* Atlanta: Centers for Disease Control and Prevention, 2005.

46. MacDonald G, Starr G, Schooley M, Yee SL, Klimowski K, Turner K. *Introduction to Program Evaluation for Comprehensive Tobacco Control Programs.* Atlanta: Centers for Disease Control and Prevention, 2001.

47. Centers for Disease Control and Prevention. *Best Practices for Comprehensive Tobacco Control Programs — October 2007.* Atlanta: U.S. Department of Health and Human Services, Centers for Disease Control and Prevention, National Center for Chronic Disease Prevention and Health Promotion, Office on Smoking and Health, 2007.

48. U.S. Department of Health and Human Services. *Ending the Tobacco Epidemic: A Tobacco Control Strategic Action Plan for the U.S. Department of Health and Human Services.* Washington: Office of the Assistant Secretary for Health, 2010.

49. Land T, Rigotti N, Levy D, Paskowsky M, Warner D, Kwass J, Wetherell L, Keithly L. A longitudinal study of Medicaid coverage for tobacco dependence treatments in Massachusetts and associated decreases in hospitalizations for cardiovascular disease. *PLoS Medicine* 2010;7(12):e1000375.

50. California Department of Health Services. California Releases New Data and Anti-Smoking Ads Targeting Diverse Populations. News Release No. 06-82, 2006; accessed: December 2, 2013.

51. Centers for Disease Control and Prevention. Vital signs: current cigarette smoking among adults aged ≥18 years with mental illness — United States, 2009–2011. *Morbidity and Mortality Weekly Report* 2013;62(05);81–7.

52. New York State Department of Health. *Cooperative Agreement Interim Progress Report.* Unpublished report submitted to CDC, 2007.

53. Centers for Disease Control and Prevention. *Best Practices for Comprehensive Tobacco Control Programs — August 1999.* Atlanta: U.S. Department of Health and Human Services, Centers for Disease Control and Prevention, National Center for Chronic Disease Prevention and Health Promotion, Office on Smoking and Health, 1999.

54. Thomas R, Perera R. School-based programmes for preventing smoking. *Cochrane Database of Systematic Reviews* 2006, Issue 3. Art. No.: CD001293. DOI: 10.1002/14651858.CD001293.pub3.

II. Mass-Reach Health Communication Interventions

Justification

Mass-reach health communication interventions can be powerful tools for preventing the initiation of tobacco use, promoting and facilitating cessation, and shaping social norms related to tobacco use.[1,2] The Community Preventive Services Task Force recommends mass-reach health communication interventions on the basis of strong evidence of effectiveness in: decreasing the prevalence of tobacco use; increasing cessation and use of available cessation services such as quitlines; and decreasing initiation of tobacco use among young people.[3]

Mass-reach health communication refers to the various means by which public health information reaches large numbers of people. The term "mass-reach" has been added to the description of health communication interventions in this edition of *Best Practices* because the available evidence suggests that the use of mass-reach vehicles, in particular television, is required to make meaningful changes in population-level awareness, knowledge, attitudes, and behaviors.[3]

Impact of Tobacco Advertising and Promotion

Billions of dollars are spent annually by tobacco companies to make tobacco use more affordable and attractive, as well as an accepted and established part of American culture.[4,5] Young people are particularly vulnerable to social and environmental influences to use tobacco. Messages and images that make tobacco use appealing to them are everywhere.[2,6] For example, youth and young adults see smoking in movies, video games, Web sites, in their social circles, and throughout the communities where they live. Tobacco marketing portrays smoking as a social norm, and young people exposed to these images are more likely to smoke. Nonsmoking adolescents exposed to tobacco advertising and promotional campaigns are significantly more likely to become young adult smokers.[2,7,8] Youth who are exposed to images of smoking in movies are more likely to smoke. Those with the most exposure to onscreen smoking imagery are about twice as likely to begin smoking as those with the least exposure.[2] Evidence also indicates that tobacco purchase and cessation behaviors among adult smokers are influenced by tobacco promotion, particularly at the point of purchase.[9–11] Because youth and adults continue to be heavily exposed to pro-tobacco media, advertising, and promotion, public education campaigns are needed to prevent tobacco use initiation and to promote cessation.

Despite the 1998 Master Settlement Agreement (MSA) between 46 states and several major tobacco companies that established restrictions on tobacco marketing and some types of outdoor advertising, tobacco product promotion remains prevalent. In 2011, tobacco companies spent more than $8.3 billion, or approximately $23 million per day, to market cigarettes in the United States;[4] this level of spending exceeded spending on tobacco prevention and control efforts by all of the states and territories by a ratio of approximately 18 to 1.[4,12] In addition, marketing expenditures for smokeless tobacco exceeded $452 million in 2011—more than double the spending in 2000.[5] Although the majority of current tobacco marketing comprises price discounts, which offset the impact of excise taxes on tobacco use, traditional tobacco company advertising and marketing spending, at more than $700 million in 2011, still far exceeds the $175 million spent on public health-sponsored antitobacco campaigns by the states and CDC.[4,5,13] Since the MSA, tobacco promotions have shifted away from traditional media (e.g., billboards and magazines) and moved toward digital media and retail outlets,[2,14–17] and tobacco companies are increasingly using tobacco product packages (e.g., shapes, colors, text) as a form of marketing.[18,19] In addition, tobacco companies are re-entering the television market as they acquire or introduce electronic cigarette (e-cigarette) products and advertise these products.[20] For example, Lorillard, Inc. acquired the e-cigarette manufacturer blu eCig® in 2012 and was among the first companies to advertise an e-cigarette product nationally on television.[21]

Tobacco advertising and promotion are real threats to public health. The 2012 Surgeon General's report stated, "The evidence is sufficient to conclude that there is a causal relationship between advertising and promotional efforts of the tobacco companies and the initiation and progression of tobacco use among young people."[2] The National Cancer Institute's (NCI's) *Monograph 19* concluded that a causal relationship exists between tobacco advertising and promotion and increased tobacco use, including both increased smoking initiation and increased per capita tobacco consumption in the population.[19] Evidence-based strategies, including mass-reach health communication interventions, are needed to counter the negative impact of tobacco industry marketing efforts and protect public health.[19]

Effectiveness of Tobacco Countermarketing

The research literature provides ample evidence that tobacco countermarketing, which is the use of commercial marketing tactics to reduce the prevalence of tobacco use, can be a valuable tool in reducing smoking.[19,22] The NCI *Monograph 19* reviewed the available literature from 1970 through 2007 and found extensive evidence that tobacco countermarketing campaigns curbed smoking initiation in youth and promoted smoking cessation in adults, particularly in the context of comprehensive tobacco control programs.[19] A 2012 review further confirmed the efficacy of mass-media campaigns in reducing smoking among adults.[23] In addition, a 2013 study found that greater exposure to tobacco control mass-media campaigns may reduce the likelihood of relapse among quitters.[24]

Media campaign research and evaluations have shown that advertising that elicits negative emotions through graphic and personal portrayals of the health consequences of tobacco use is especially effective in motivating smokers to quit.[19,23,25] There is also evidence that this kind of approach to advertising messages reduces tobacco use among youth and young adults.[2,26] CDC's *Tips From Former Smokers (Tips)* campaign, the first federally funded, nationwide, paid-media tobacco education campaign in the United States, is an example of this approach. The first *Tips* campaign was conducted during March–June 2012 and featured former smokers talking about their experiences and their families' experiences living with diseases caused by smoking and secondhand smoke exposure.[27] In addition to a comprehensive earned media component, the *Tips* campaign included advertising on national and local television, local radio, online media, and billboards as well as in movie theaters, transit venues, and print media. A subsequent evaluation of *Tips* found that an estimated 1.6 million smokers attempted to quit smoking because of the campaign and that more than 100,000 of them would likely quit smoking permanently.[26] Additionally, the 2012 *Tips* campaign and a subsequent 2013 *Tips* campaign resulted in immediate and significant increases in state quitline call volumes, which rapidly declined to baseline levels upon completion of these campaigns.[26,27]

There have been fewer studies examining the effectiveness of tobacco countermarketing campaigns among population subgroups that bear a disproportionate burden of tobacco-related disease and death. However, some studies have assessed the potential differential impact of mass-media campaigns by socioeconomic status (SES). A 2012 review found evidence to suggest that general-population campaigns may be effective for encouraging quitting in low SES smokers if the campaigns have sufficient reach, frequency, and duration.[23] A 2012 study in New York state found increased quit attempts among both the general population and low-SES groups who were exposed to strongly emotional and graphic antismoking advertisements.[25]

Over the past decade, states have remained an important source of innovative countermarketing content; however, many have also found that they can save time, money, and the risks associated with new advertisement development by adapting existing advertisements from other states, cities, national governmental agencies, or other countries. For example, New York City has used advertisements from Australia, England, Massachusetts, California, and Minnesota; Florida has used advertisements from Australia, California, Washington State, and New York City; and Minnesota has used advertisements from Canada, California, Vermont, Ohio, Arizona, and CDC.[28] Many of the advertisements were found in CDC's Media Campaign Resource Center (MCRC) database.[28]

In addition to the importance of effective messaging strategies, research from many sources shows that tobacco countermarketing campaigns must have sufficient reach, frequency, and duration to be successful.[24,27,29-31] A key goal for tobacco control campaigns is to reach a defined target audience with attention-getting messages in the most efficient and effective way possible. Media buying, which typically includes how placements are purchased, the channels selected, and how the budget is allocated across channels, is an integral part of an overall strategy.

Evidence also suggests that earned media, which is the process of securing free news placements in a variety of media outlets through dedicated efforts to communicate key messages, can contribute to tobacco countermarketing campaign effectiveness. Local and statewide earned media campaigns have been shown to effectively support key tobacco control goals, including increasing calls to a state quitline, influencing smoking knowledge, attitudes, and behavior among youth, and implementing changes in local tobacco control policy.[32-35]

Digital media, including electronic delivery of information via Web sites, mobile applications, and social networking sites, are emerging and promising vehicles for reaching and influencing key target audiences. However, there is not yet sufficient evidence to draw conclusions or to make formal recommendations on the efficacy or ideal use of these media at this time. The measurement and evaluation of digital media interventions are critical to help build an evidence base, to gauge their effectiveness, and to optimize future digital media interventions. Given that the tobacco industry is allocating significant funding to these media,[4,5] use of digital media is likely a promising area for states to consider.

Recommendations

An effective state mass-reach health communication intervention delivers strategic, culturally appropriate, and high-impact messages via sustained and adequately funded campaigns that are integrated into a comprehensive state tobacco control program effort. Typically, effective health communication interventions and countermarketing strategies employ a wide range of efforts, including:[22]

- Paid television, radio, out-of-home (e.g., billboards, transit), print, and digital advertising at the state and local levels

- Media advocacy through public relations/earned media efforts (e.g., press releases/conferences, social media, and local events), which are often timed to coincide with holidays, heritage months, and health observances

- Health promotion activities, such as working with health care professionals and other partners and promoting quitlines

- Efforts to reduce or replace tobacco industry sponsorship and promotions as well as to decrease movie smoking imagery

Innovations in health communication interventions include the ability to target and engage specific audiences through multiple communication channels, such as online video, mobile Web, and smartphone and tablet applications (apps). Social media platforms, such as Twitter and Facebook, have facilitated improvements in how messages are developed, fostered, and disseminated in order to better communicate with target audiences and allow for relevant, credible messages to be shared more broadly within the target audiences' social circles. However, these platforms are complements to, not substitutes for, traditional mass media. Because data on the contribution of digital media efforts to reaching tobacco countermarketing campaign goals are still emerging, evaluation of digital media efforts can help determine effectiveness and establish an evidence base.[22]

Behavior theory, audience insight research, pre-testing of campaign materials, and surveillance and evaluation are grounded in communication science and are used to develop interventions that target specific audiences with messages that can change awareness, knowledge, attitudes, and behaviors. Examples of these audiences include adult tobacco users, youth, and high-risk populations such as members of the lesbian, gay, bisexual, and transgender (LGBT) communities, those with lower socioeconomic status, and certain races such as American Indians. These methods are often used to identify key strategies, influential messages, and the most effective communication channels and media options to reach specific audiences. However, ensuring that messages resonate with specific population subgroups does not require that unique materials be developed for each audience. Evidence has confirmed that strong ads, such as those that graphically or emotionally portray the serious consequences of smoking, resonate well with a wide variety of audiences.[19,23] Advertising concepts and advertisements can be tested among specific target audiences to ensure that they communicate persuasively, and media buying can be tailored, when feasible, to ensure appropriate reach of those audiences.

Effective media planning works within the total framework of a mass-reach health communication campaign's goals. For an overall campaign, it is estimated that advertisements should reach 75% to 85% of the target audience each quarter of the year, with a minimum average per quarter of 1,200 gross rating points (GRPs) during the introduction of a campaign and a minimum average of 800 GRPs per quarter thereafter.[22,23,29,36] GRPs track the total reach and frequency of the campaign. A campaign is expected to run at least 3 to 6 months to achieve awareness of the issue, 6 to 12 months to influence attitudes, and 12 to 18 months to influence behavior,[22,29] although some campaigns, including CDC's *Tips* campaign, have influenced behavior within a 3-month time frame.[26,27] Campaigns need to overcome pro-tobacco marketing influences; thus, it is important to set reasonable expectations of effectiveness. In addition, campaigns must run as continuously as possible because their impact can diminish over a relatively short time period.[26,27,37–39] For more information regarding the media planning process, consult CDC's countermarketing manual, *Designing and Implementing an Effective Tobacco Countermarketing Campaign*.[22]

The experiences of many states, including New York, California, Florida, Massachusetts, and Minnesota; the national organization Legacy (formerly the American Legacy Foundation); and CDC emphasize that message content of tobacco control campaigns is very important. Messages that elicit strong emotional response, such as personal testimonials and viscerally negative content, produce stronger and more consistent effects on audience recall, knowledge, beliefs and quitting behaviors.[2,22,25,26,40] Aggressive state and national countermarketing campaigns that have more directly confronted the tobacco industry's marketing tactics have also demonstrated effectiveness, but have often become targets for budget cuts.[41–43]

Resources such as CDC's countermarketing manual and the MCRC database can be used to develop effective communications plans and to acquire effective advertisements cost efficiently.[22,28] The countermarketing manual is a toolkit with chapters on all major aspects of campaign development, and MCRC is a clearinghouse of tobacco-related media campaign materials produced by states and other organizations that other states can adapt and reuse. Evidence suggests that it is not necessary to develop new advertising,[44–46] particularly considering the availability of existing advertisements in the MCRC—many of which have been used with very effective results.[28] Typically, new advertising should be developed only when a campaign objective is unique enough that existing advertisements may not address it, when a campaign needs to publicize a local event (e.g., a quitting program or implementation of a new smokefree law), or when another unique situation arises.

Comprehensive earned media efforts are an essential part of the strategic plan, regardless of the size of one's media campaign budget, but especially when funds are limited. Additionally, each major campaign element and activity should have an earned media component. Although paid media benefits from the ability to control the message and the placement, news media coverage is important because it can help set the public agenda, influence what people are talking about, and further broaden and add credibility to paid messages. Examples of earned media tactics include: establishing relationships with journalists to become a trusted, responsive, and knowledgeable resource; issuing press releases; scheduling editorial board briefings; holding events to generated media coverage; writing letters to the editor; and training spokespeople for interviews.[22,28,32–34]

In addition to providing sufficient reach, frequency, and duration, effective media and mass-reach health communication intervention efforts will benefit from the activities identified in the following box.

Beneficial Activities for Effective Media and Mass-Reach Health Communication Intervention Efforts

- Audience insight research to determine the current knowledge, attitudes, and behaviors of target audiences, as well as the motivations and behavioral theory that can best influence change among specific audiences.

- Formative research to identify promising messages and concepts.

- Formative evaluation to pretest campaign materials to ensure that they are clear, credible, and persuasive and that they motivate the audience to change their attitudes and behaviors.

- Surveillance to understand pro-tobacco messaging, media placements, and marketing tactics.

- Local media promotion, event sponsorships, and other community collaboration tie-ins to support and reinforce the statewide campaign, increase awareness about policies that protect and promote health, and shift social norms related to tobacco use.

- Digital technologies, such as text/SMS messaging, social media, Web sites, and blogs to generate messages that can be further disseminated by the target audience.

- Process and outcome evaluation of a comprehensive communication effort, as well as specific evaluations of new and innovative approaches, including the use of digital media.

- Promotion of available services, including the state's telephone cessation quitline number or the quitline portal numbers (1-800-QUIT-NOW, 1-855-DÉJELO-YA), as well as quitting Web sites and social media pages.

Achieving Equity to Reduce Tobacco-Related Disparities

Recognition of, and sensitivity to, diverse audiences is critically important in tobacco control mass-reach health communications campaigns, particularly to address disparities in tobacco use and corresponding inequities in tobacco-related health outcomes across population groups. The experiences of multiple states and CDC have shown that mass-reach health communication campaign funds can be efficiently and effectively used to reach and influence populations with the greatest tobacco-related burden through carefully-planned formative research that determines which messages and approaches resonate powerfully across diverse audiences, as well as thoughtful media placement that reaches key audiences where and when they are most receptive to the messages.

Television advertisements that are not tailored by audience segment are frequently used by state tobacco control programs in an effort to ensure the broad and consistent delivery of key messages. This approach is supported by evidence suggesting that there are some universally strong messages for tobacco prevention education advertisements, such as the serious negative effects of smoking on the body and the emotional impact on family members, and that these types of messages are effective across a broad spectrum of geographies and populations without requiring significant tailoring.[19,23,47] However, it is still important to consider and address audience diversity when developing or selecting advertisements. For example, testimonial advertisements could feature individuals of varied sexes, ages, race/ethnicities, sexual orientations, gender identities, or other population characteristics. At the national level, CDC's *Tips* campaign featured testimonials of former smokers from multiple population groups with high rates of tobacco use.[27]

Some state tobacco control programs also tailor media buys to reach specific audience segments within general-population campaigns. For example, certain population subgroups may be more likely to listen to radio, while others may be more likely to read language-specific print materials or to engage in social media. States can use these media channels to cost efficiently supplement television placements. For example, to reach low-SES male audiences, North Carolina placed an advertisement in a NASCAR publication and distributed earplugs with the state's quitline number at the race. Similarly, New York purchased placement on a sports cable network and used baseball-themed advertisements from Florida and Massachusetts. To reach American Indians and Alaska Natives, CDC purchased placements on radio networks and regional print publications targeted to these audiences.

When planning and developing a mass-reach health communication campaign, the most critical considerations are that the messages resonate effectively with each priority audience and that the tailored media placements help ensure that each key audience notices and internalizes those messages. Taking into account these considerations should ultimately help increase the likelihood that the messages lead to meaningful changes in tobacco-related knowledge, attitudes, and behaviors.

Budget

Mass-reach health communication efforts must be adequately funded, sustained over time, and integrated with other program activities in order to counter tobacco industry marketing, reduce tobacco use initiation, increase cessation, and reduce exposure to secondhand smoke.

Campaigns of longer duration and higher reach and frequency are associated with greater declines in smoking rates.[2,22,23,48] Future funding for national campaigns sponsored by CDC, Legacy, and other organizations remains uncertain, and even if federal mass-media campaign efforts are conducted during some years, they are not sufficient alone and should not take the place of state-level media campaigns. Therefore, states may want to plan to provide the primary budget for mass-reach health communication interventions to ensure broad population-level exposure to messages that address the goals of a comprehensive tobacco control program. The three major content areas of these messages include:

- Motivating tobacco users to quit
- Protecting people from the harms of secondhand smoke
- Transforming social norms to prevent tobacco use initiation

Budget recommendations should be sufficient to conduct mass-reach health communication campaigns in the state's major media markets addressing these three key content areas. Evidence suggests that if proven message strategies are used, such as personal and graphic portrayals of the negative health consequences of tobacco use, the same advertisements can be effective among both youth and adults,[2,19] thus maximizing the impact of limited funds. Funds can be competitively awarded to firms that understand a state's media markets, have experience in reaching culturally diverse audiences, have the ability to conduct market research and surveillance of counter-marketing efforts, and exhibit a willingness to review existing advertising before recommending that new advertising be developed. Additional guidance on selecting contractors for health communication interventions is available in *Designing and Implementing an Effective Tobacco Countermarketing Campaign.*[22]

Budget estimates for funding mass-reach health communication interventions are generally based on the *Best Practices—2007* funding formula, but the estimates have been revised based upon more recent state and national experiences. These evidence-based levels of media presence were used to calculate the *minimum* and *recommended* levels of spending (see Appendix A for more details).

The *minimum* budget level assumes that three campaigns are conducted each year to address the following goals: 1) motivating smokers to quit; 2) protecting people from the harms of secondhand smoke exposure; and 3) transforming social norms to prevent tobacco use initiation, with a delivery of an average of 1,200 GRPs per quarter for either one of the cessation or secondhand smoke campaigns (assumes it is an introductory campaign and, thus, requires higher levels) and a delivery of an average of 800 GRPs for each of the other two campaigns. The *minimum* budget level also assumes a 20% reduction in costs to account for efficiencies in message communication and media negotiation (reduced rates or bonus placements) that would be expected when conducting three campaigns simultaneously. The *recommended* budget level assumes delivery of campaigns with the same overall goals, with an average of 1,600 GRPs per quarter for one of the cessation or secondhand smoke campaigns and 1,200 GRPs per quarter for the other two campaigns, and a 20% reduction in costs based on message and media negotiation efficiencies.

This range of funding was applied to states according to the cost and complexity of their media markets, in part measured by the coverage provided by a state's designated market areas (DMAs). State-level cost estimates for buying televised air time in all 210 U.S. DMAs in 2014 were acquired by CDC in May 2013. States with counties that fall outside their primary DMAs may need to consider purchasing media in a neighboring state or using other vehicles, such as digital, in order to reach 75% to 85% of the target audience. Also, budgeting for cost-effective media campaigns is more complicated for states having media markets that share major metropolitan areas with neighboring states, so such states may need to rely more on local vehicles (digital, out-of-home, newsprint, radio) and less on broadcast television to limit spending to reasonable levels. However, those placements may not easily translate to GRP levels.

It is important to note that the *recommended* level of media investment is for media placement only. Because they vary significantly across states, the following costs were not included in the budget estimates: advertising agency and media planning firm fees; audience insight research; pretesting of materials; advertising development and production; and talent fees.

In addition, the more campaigns a state conducts, the more staffing will be required. Although the *Infrastructure, Administrative, and Management* chapter of this report provides general funding levels for staffing, additional funds will be needed to support three unique multimedia campaigns. Also, additional funds may be needed to tailor the campaign to specific population groups, especially to ensure language appropriateness, through the use of unique messages, materials, or media vehicles. However, states can lower advertising development costs by using existing television, radio, print, and outdoor advertisements from CDC's MCRC.[28] Also, alternative forms of communication—such as direct mail, Web sites, blogs, social media and text messaging, and working through health care providers, other government organizations, and the news media—can extend the reach and frequency of messages, as can recruiting audiences to produce or adapt, place, and promote messages themselves through social media and other digital technologies.

In the event that available funding for mass-reach health communication interventions exceeds *minimum* levels and approaches *recommended* levels, state programs may want to consider allocating resources for elements related to the creation of their own advertisements, including audience insight research and advertisement development and production. It is important to note that these funding levels are general; thus, states may have to tailor certain factors—such as number of goals, campaigns conducted, and target audiences—to their unique situations.

References

1. U.S. Department of Health and Human Services. *Reducing Tobacco Use: A Report of the Surgeon General.* Atlanta: U.S. Department of Health and Human Services, Centers for Disease Control and Prevention, National Center for Chronic Disease Prevention and Health Promotion, Office on Smoking and Health, 2000.

2. U.S. Department of Health and Human Services. *Preventing Tobacco Use Among Youth and Young Adults: A Report of the Surgeon General.* Atlanta: U.S. Department of Health and Human Services, Centers for Disease Control and Prevention, National Center for Chronic Disease Prevention and Health Promotion, Office on Smoking and Health, 2012.

3. Guide to Community Preventive Services. Reducing Tobacco Use and Secondhand Smoke Exposure: Mass-Reach Health Communication Interventions; <http://www.thecommunityguide.org/tobacco/massreach.html>; accessed: December 2, 2013.

4. Federal Trade Commission. Federal Trade Commission Cigarette Report for 2011; <http://www.ftc.gov/os/2013/05/130521cigarettereport.pdf>; accessed: December 2, 2013.

5. Federal Trade Commission. Federal Trade Commission Smokeless Tobacco Report for 2011; <http://www.ftc.gov/os/2013/05/130521smokelesstobaccoreport.pdf>; accessed: December 2, 2013.

6. Charlesworth A, Glantz SA. Tobacco and the movie industry. *Clinics in Occupational and Environmental Medicine* 2006;5(1):73–84.

7. Gilpin EA, White MM, Messer K, Pierce JP. Receptivity to tobacco advertising and promotions among young adolescents as a predictor of established smoking in young adulthood. *American Journal of Public Health* 2007;97(8):1489–95.

8. Lovato C, Watts A, Stead LF. Impact of tobacco advertising and promotion on increasing adolescent smoking behaviours. *Cochrane Database of Systematic Reviews* 2011, Issue 10. Art. No.: CD003439. DOI: 10.1002/14651858.CD003439.pub2.

9. Carter OB, Mills BW, Donovan RJ. The effect of retail cigarette pack displays on unplanned purchases: results from immediate postpurchase interviews. *Tobacco Control* 2009;18(3):218–21.

10. Clattenburg EJ, Elff JL, Apelberg BJ. Unplanned cigarette purchases and tobacco point of sale advertising: a potential barrier to smoking cessation. *Tobacco Control* 2013;22(6):376–81.

11. Germain D, McCarthy M. Smoker sensitivity to retail tobacco displays and quitting: a cohort study. *Addiction* 2010;105(1):159–63.

12. Campaign for Tobacco-Free Kids. Spending vs. Tobacco Company Marketing; <http://www.tobaccofreekids.org/content/what_we_do/state_local_issues/settlement/FY2013/10.%20State%20Tobacco%20Prevention%20Spending%20vs.%20Tob.%20Co.%20Marketing%2011-27-12.pdf>; accessed: December 2, 2013.

13. Chaloupka, F, Huang J. *State Tobacco Control Expenditure Data: 2008–2011.* Chicago: Health Policy Center, Institute for Health Research and Policy, University of Illinois–Chicago, 2013.

14. Freeman B. New media and tobacco control. *Tobacco Control* 2012; 21(2):139–44.

15. Wakefield MA, Terry-McElrath YM, Chaloupka FJ, Barker DC, Slater SJ, Clark PI, Giovino GA. Tobacco industry marketing at point of purchase after the 1998 MSA billboard advertising ban. *American Journal of Public Health* 2002;92(6):937–40.

16. Feighery EC, Schleicher NC, Boley Cruz T, Unger JB. An examination of trends in amount and type of cigarette advertising and sales promotions in California stores, 2002–2005. *Tobacco Control* 2008;17(2):93–8.

17. Loomis BR, Farrelly MC, Nonnemaker JM, Mann NH. Point of purchase cigarette promotions before and after the Master Settlement Agreement: exploring retail scanner data. *Tobacco Control* 2006;15(2):140–2.

18. Moodie C, Hastings G. Tobacco packaging as promotion. *Tobacco Control* 2010;(19):168–70.

19. National Cancer Institute. *The Role of the Media in Promoting and Reducing Tobacco Use.* Tobacco Control Monograph No. 19. Bethesda (MD): U.S. Department of Health and Human Services, Public Health Service, National Institutes of Health, National Cancer Institute, 2008. NIH Publication No. 07-6242.

20. King BA, Alam S, Promoff G, Arrazola R, Dube SR. Awareness and ever use of electronic cigarettes among U.S. adults, 2010–2011. *Nicotine & Tobacco Research* 2013;15(9):1623–7.

21. Internet Movie Database. Demo Reel (Blu E-cig National TV Commercial); <http://www.imdb.com/video/demo_reel/vi2066392089/>; accessed: December 2, 2013.

22. Centers for Disease Control and Prevention. *Designing and Implementing an Effective Tobacco Countermarketing Campaign*. Atlanta: U.S. Department of Health and Human Services, Centers for Disease Control and Prevention, National Center for Chronic Disease Prevention and Health Promotion, Office on Smoking and Health, 2003.

23. Durkin S, Brennan E, Wakefield M. Mass media campaigns to promote smoking cessation among adults: an integrative review. *Tobacco Control* 2012;21(2):127–38.

24. Wakefield MA, Bowe SJ, Durkin SJ, Yong HH, Spittal MJ, Simpson JA, Borland R. Does tobacco-control mass media campaign exposure prevent relapse among recent quitters? *Nicotine & Tobacco Research* 2013;15(2):385–92.

25. Farrelly MC, Duke JC, Davis KC, Nonnemaker JM, Kamyab K, Willett JG, Juster HR. Promotion of smoking cessation with emotional and/or graphic antismoking advertising. *American Journal of Preventive Medicine* 2012;43(5):475–82.

26. McAfee T, Davis KC, Alexander RL, Pechacek TF, Bunnel R. Effect of the first federally funded US antismoking national media campaign. *Lancet* 2013;382(9909):2003-11.

27. Centers for Disease Control and Prevention. Increases in quitline calls and smoking cessation website visitors during a national tobacco education campaign — March 19–June10, 2012. *Morbidity and Mortality Weekly Report* 2012;61(34):667–70.

28. Centers for Disease Control and Prevention. Media Campaign Resource Center Online Database; <http://www.cdc.gov/tobacco/media_campaigns/index.htm>; accessed: December 2, 2013.

29. Schar E, Gutierrez K, Murphy-Hoefer R, Nelson DE. *Tobacco Use Prevention Media Campaigns: Lessons Learned from Youth in Nine Countries*. Atlanta: U.S. Department of Health and Human Services, Centers for Disease Control and Prevention, National Center for Chronic Disease Prevention and Health Promotion, Office on Smoking and Health, 2006.

30. Terry-McElrath Y, Wakefield M, Ruel E, Balch GI, Emery S, Szczypka G, et al. The effect of antismoking advertisement executional characteristics on youth comprehension, appraisal, recall, and engagement. *Journal of Health Communication* 2005;10:127–43.

31. Terry-McElrath YM, Emery S, Wakefield MA, O'Malley PM, Szczypka G, Johnston LD. Effects of tobacco-related media campaigns on smoking among 20-30-year-old adults: longitudinal data from the USA. *Tobacco Control* 2013;22(1):38–45.

32. Sheffer MA, Redmond LA, Kobinsky KH, Keller PA, McAfee T, Fiore MC. Creating a perfect storm to increase consumer demand for Wisconsin's Tobacco Quitline. *American Journal of Preventive Medicine* 2010;38(3 Suppl):343S–346S.

33. Smith KC, Wakefield MA, Terry-McElrath Y, Chaloupka FJ, Flay B, Johnston L, Saba A, Siebel C. Relation between newspaper coverage of tobacco issues and smoking attitudes and behaviour among American teens. *Tobacco Control* 2008;17(1):17–24.

34. Dunlop SM, Romer D. Relation between newspaper coverage of 'light' cigarette litigation and beliefs about 'lights' among American adolescents and young adults: the impact on risk perceptions and quitting intentions. *Tobacco Control* 2010;19(4):267–73.

35. Niederdeppe J, Farrelly MC, Wenter D. Media advocacy, tobacco control policy change and teen smoking in Florida. *Tobacco Control* 2007;16(1):47–52.

36. White VM, Durkin SJ, Coomber K, Wakefield MA. What is the role of tobacco control advertising intensity and duration in reducing adolescent smoking prevalence? Findings from 16 years of tobacco control mass media advertising in Australia. *Tobacco Control* 2013 Aug 29. Epub ahead of print. DOI: 10.1136/tobaccocontrol-2012-050945.

37. Wakefield MA, Durkin S, Spittal MJ, Siahpush M, Scollo M, Simpson JA, Chapman S, White V, Hill D. Impact of tobacco control policies and mass media campaigns on monthly adult smoking prevalence. *American Journal of Public Health* 2008;98(8):1443–50.

38. Dietz NA, Westphal L, Arheart KL, Lee DJ, Huang Y, Sly DF, Davila E. Changes in youth cigarette use following the dismantling of an antitobacco media campaign in Florida. *Preventing Chronic Disease* 2010;7(3):A65.

39. Centers for Disease Control and Prevention. Effect of ending an antitobacco youth campaign on adolescent susceptibility to cigarette smoking — Minnesota, 2002–2003. *Morbidity and Mortality Weekly Report* 2004;53(14):301–4.

40. Wakefield M, Loken B, Hornik R. Use of mass media campaigns to change health behavior. *Lancet* 2010;376:1261–71.

41. Ibrahim JK, Glantz SA. The rise and fall of tobacco control media campaigns, 1967–2006. *American Journal of Public Health* 2007;97(8):1383–96.

42. Farrelly MC, Nonnemaker J, Davis KC, Hussin A. The influence of the national truth campaign on smoking initiation. *American Journal of Preventive Medicine* 2009;36(5):379–84.

43. Holtgrave DR, Wunderink KA, Vallone DM, Healton CG. Cost–utility analysis of the national truth campaign to prevent youth smoking. *American Journal of Preventive Medicine* 2009;36(5):385–8.

44. Cotter T, Perez D, Dunlop S, Hung WT, Dessaix A, Bishop JF. The case for recycling and adapting anti-tobacco mass media campaigns. *Tobacco Control* 2010;19(6):514–7.

45. Wakefield M, Bayly M, Durkin S, Cotter T, Millin S, Warne C, International Anti-Tobacco Advertisement Rating Study Team. Smokers' responses to television advertisements about the serious harms of tobacco use: pre-testing results from 10 low- to middle-income countries. *Tobacco Control* 2013;22(1):24–31.

46. Perl R, Stebenkova L, Morozova I, Murukutla N, Kochetova V, Kotov A, Voylokova T, Baskakova J. Mass media campaigns within reach: effective efforts with limited resources in Russia's capital city. *Tobacco Control* 2011;20(6):439–41.

47. Durkin SJ, Biener L, Wakefield MA. Effects of different types of antismoking ads on reducing disparities in smoking cessation among socioeconomic subgroups. *American Journal of Public Health* 2009;99(12):2217–23.

48. Centers for Disease Control and Prevention. *Best Practices for Comprehensive Tobacco Control Programs — October 2007.* Atlanta: U.S. Department of Health and Human Services, Centers for Disease Control and Prevention, National Center for Chronic Disease Prevention and Health Promotion, Office on Smoking and Health, 2007.

III. Cessation Interventions

Justification

Rationale

Promoting cessation is a core component of a comprehensive state tobacco control program's efforts to reduce tobacco use.[1,2] Encouraging and helping tobacco users to quit is the quickest approach to reducing tobacco-related disease, death, and health care costs.[3] Quitting smoking has immediate and long-term health benefits.[4] Although quitting smoking at any age is beneficial, smokers who quit by the time they are 35 to 44 years of age avoid most of the risk of dying from a smoking-related disease.[5]

Population-wide interventions that change societal environments and norms related to tobacco use—including increases in the unit price of tobacco products, comprehensive smokefree policies, and hard-hitting media campaigns—increase tobacco cessation by motivating tobacco users to quit and making it easier for them to do so.[1-3,6,7] Offering cessation assistance to smokers who attempt to quit in response to these interventions maximizes the impact of these interventions on cessation, while countering the perception that they are punitive.[1-3,6-8]

Guiding Principles

Population-wide cessation efforts—specifically, policy, systems, or environmental changes—are most efficient and effective at reaching many people.[1,2,6,8] Systems changes within health care organizations complement interventions in state and community settings by institutionalizing sustainable approaches that support individual behavior change.[1,6,8] As in other areas of tobacco control, policy and/or systems approaches support healthy behaviors at both the individual and the societal or institutional levels.[1,6,8]

Although it is appropriate and necessary for comprehensive state tobacco control programs to fund and provide certain cessation treatment services (i.e., to directly deliver cessation counseling and medications through population-based approaches such as state quitlines) to certain populations, particularly groups that would otherwise not have access to these services (e.g. the uninsured), the programs' focus should remain on population-level, strategic efforts to reconfigure policies and systems in ways that normalize quitting and that institutionalize tobacco use screening and intervention within medical care.[1,6,8]

State tobacco control programs can educate private and public health care systems, health insurers, and employers on the importance of assuming responsibility for, and covering the costs of, providing cessation services to their members and employees.[1] States can also monitor and leverage provisions in the Affordable Care Act that require new private health plans and state Medicaid programs to expand coverage of evidence-based tobacco use cessation treatments.[9] The Affordable Care Act and the Health Information Technology for Economic and Clinical Health Act, which gave rise to the Meaningful Use of Electronic Health Records Incentive Program, provide states with a unique opportunity to focus cessation efforts on promoting and supporting the implementation of policies and systems within health care organizations and health insurers that support cessation, and also offer eligible providers and hospitals federal funding to adopt electronic health records and use them in ways that can support improvements in the delivery of clinical preventive services, including tobacco dependence treatment.

Such policies and systems have the potential to dramatically increase the delivery of evidence-based cessation interventions, thus making them more widely available and accessible. Cessation services directly provided or funded by a comprehensive state tobacco control program are best focused on populations that lack access to these services through other channels, such as the uninsured and the underinsured.[10] In addition, state programs may perform some functions that are most efficiently handled at a centralized level, such as tagging mass-media advertisements with a phone number or Web site where individuals can obtain or be referred to basic cessation services.

Population quit rates are determined by two factors: (1) the number of quit attempts, which includes the number of smokers who try to quit, and the number of times they make a quit attempt; and (2) the odds that smokers who try to quit will succeed in doing so.[11] It is important that state efforts to increase population quit rates strive to increase both quit attempts and quit success, and attempt to strike a balance between the reach and intensity of interventions.[1,11] State tobacco control programs play an important role in implementing interventions such as hard-hitting media campaigns that motivate smokers to quit, as well as ensuring that smokers who want help quitting, but who lack adequate cessation coverage, have access to effective cessation assistance and know how to obtain it.

Two-thirds to three-quarters of smokers who try to quit do not use any evidence-based cessation counseling or medications.[12,13] Smokers improve their odds of successfully quitting when they use these treatments.[14] It is important for state cessation initiatives to make smokers aware of this fact and to ensure that cessation treatments are readily available through health care systems and providers, state telephone quitlines, and other community-based cessation resources.[1] This message can be communicated without implying that smokers cannot quit successfully without using cessation treatments, so as not to lessen the impact of tobacco education campaigns on increasing quit attempts.[15,16]

An Altered Landscape

The cessation landscape has changed considerably since *Best Practices—2007* as a result of the following developments:

- Publication of an updated version of the Public Health Services Clinical Practice Guideline, *Treating Tobacco Use and Dependence*, in 2008
- Enactment of the Patient Protection and Affordable Care Act
- Implementation of the Meaningful Use initiative
- Widespread adoption of electronic health records
- Creation of the Centers for Medicare and Medicaid Innovation
- Introduction of new voluntary Joint Commission hospital cessation performance measures
- Increasing shift to managed care plans in state Medicaid programs
- Changes in the organization of private health care
- Increased emphasis on establishing linkages between public health interventions and clinical interventions
- Introduction of the national tobacco education media campaign, *Tips From Former Smokers,* conducted by CDC

These changes have presented significant new opportunities to expand cessation coverage, institutionalize tobacco use screening and interventions within health care systems, and increase the availability and use of evidence-based cessation treatments.

Three Major Goals

Comprehensive state tobacco control program cessation activities should focus on three broad goals:

- Promoting health systems change
- Expanding insurance coverage and utilization of proven cessation treatments
- Supporting state quitline capacity

Promoting Health Systems Change

The health care system provides multiple opportunities for motivating and helping smokers to quit.[6,8,14,17] More than 80% of smokers see a physician every year,[18] and most smokers want and expect their physicians to talk to them about quitting smoking and are receptive to their physicians' advice.[14] Tobacco dependence treatment is both clinically effective and highly cost-effective, and results in reduced health care costs, increased productivity, and reduced absenteeism.[14]

Effective tobacco cessation interventions advance the goals of national and state health care reform efforts to improve health care, to improve health, and to reduce health care costs. Health systems change involves institutionalizing cessation interventions in health care systems and integrating these interventions into routine clinical care.[6,8,14,17] This increases the likelihood that health care providers will consistently screen patients for tobacco use and intervene with patients who use tobacco, thus increasing cessation and making evidence-based tobacco dependence treatment the standard of care.[14,17,19] When a health system seeks to intervene with every tobacco user at every visit,[14] it can substantially and rapidly increase cessation.[14,17,19]

State efforts to promote health systems change involve working with health care systems and organizations to fully integrate tobacco dependence treatment into the clinical workflow.[6,8,14,17,19] The goal is to ensure that every patient is screened for tobacco use, their tobacco use status is documented, and patients who use tobacco are advised to quit.[6,8,14,17,19] This is followed by offering the patient cessation medication (unless contraindicated), counseling, and assistance, as well as arranging follow-up contact either on-site or through referrals to the state quitline or other community resources.[6,8,14,17,19,20] This approach has been summarized as the "5 A's": (1) ask about tobacco use; (2) advise to quit; (3) assess willingness to make a quit attempt; (4) assist in the quit attempt; and (5) arrange follow-up.[14]

One way to increase the use of this approach is through provider reminder systems, which prompt health care providers to screen and intervene with patients around tobacco use and increase provider delivery of cessation advice.[6,14] Consistent screening and delivery of cessation interventions are also facilitated by assigning multiple members of the health care team (e.g., medical assistants, physician assistants, nurses, and physicians) clearly identified roles in this area.[14]

State tobacco control programs can promote health systems change in multiple ways. For example, state governments provide health care coverage to Medicaid enrollees and state employees. States also regulate or otherwise interact with the health insurance market. These roles provide opportunities to improve health systems approaches to tobacco use prevention and cessation. In addition, state tobacco control programs can educate health care decision makers about the health and economic burden imposed by tobacco use and the evidence base for clinical cessation interventions, including the cost-effectiveness and return on investment of these interventions.[1,21,22] State tobacco control programs can also offer technical assistance to help health care organizations and providers measure the implementation of health systems changes and the impact of these changes on outcomes in their patient populations using data from electronic health records, insurance claims, and other sources.

State programs can further support health systems change by carrying out academic detailing initiatives.[21,22] This involves providing technical assistance to health care organizations and providers in implementing health systems changes that institutionalize tobacco use screening and intervention, including referrals to the state quitline.[20-24] The technical assistance is typically provided in-person in the health care setting by trained personnel.[21,22] Studies of academic detailing initiatives have found that they have the potential to increase: use of the "5 As";[25,26] frequency of tobacco cessation counseling;[27] appropriate use of cessation medications;[27] and fax referrals to quitlines.[20-24]

Under the Meaningful Use initiative, the Centers for Medicare and Medicaid Services is making substantial financial incentives available to eligible providers and hospitals to migrate from paper to electronic health records in order to improve health care and health care outcomes.[28] When electronic health records are implemented in a way that explicitly incorporates tobacco dependence treatment as part of a broader process of health systems change, they can serve as a powerful provider reminder system, prompting providers to screen their patients for, and intervene on, tobacco use by embedding prompts, language, and documentation within the records themselves, and helping to seamlessly integrate these steps into the clinical workflow.[29-33] The implementation of electronic health records with a cessation component can have an even greater impact if it is coupled with training and technical assistance to all members of the health care team.[32,33]

Electronic health records can also make it easier for providers to refer patients to state quitlines, counseling within the health organization, and community-based cessation programs, especially when these referrals can be made electronically.[20,30-32] Several provisions of the initial stages of Meaningful Use require electronic health records to capture identification of and intervention with patients who use tobacco and require providers to report on these measures in order to receive financial rewards.[8,20]

Health care organizations that have implemented electronic health records in combination with other health systems changes are able to achieve levels of 80% or higher for both screening and intervention, with additional improvement possible.[19] State tobacco control programs can seek opportunities to leverage the implementation of electronic health records by working with large health care systems to integrate tobacco dependence treatment into their workflows.[33] Electronic health records can also be used to monitor provider performance for purposes of feedback, recognition, and rewards at the organization and/or provider levels, as well as to conduct surveillance of tobacco-related measures.[19,30]

Finally, new hospital performance measures implemented by the Joint Commission in January 2012 expand and strengthen previous Joint Commission measures by calling on hospitals to provide cessation interventions to all tobacco users, not just those with specific diagnoses, and by expanding the scope of these interventions.[34-36] State tobacco control programs can work with the health care sector to encourage hospitals to adopt these voluntary cessation measures and can provide technical assistance with implementation.[36]

Sample State Activities: Promoting Health Systems Change

- Build and maintain relationships with large health care systems and key stakeholders in the health care sector, and educate them about the feasibility and health and economic benefits of integrating tobacco dependence treatment into their clinical workflows.

- Conduct academic detailing initiatives to provide technical assistance to health care organizations and providers in implementing health systems changes that institutionalize tobacco use screening and intervention, including promoting referrals to the state quitline.

- Collaborate with health care systems, regional extension centers, and other stakeholders to integrate tobacco dependence treatment into electronic health records and workflows.

- Leverage data from electronic health records, insurance claims, and other sources for surveillance/evaluation of the implementation and outcomes of health systems change cessation interventions.

Expanding Insurance Coverage and Utilization of Proven Cessation Treatments

Expanding cessation insurance coverage increases the number of smokers who attempt to quit, use evidence-based cessation treatments, and successfully quit by removing cost and administrative barriers that prevent smokers from accessing cessation counseling and medications.[6,14,17,37]

Expanding cessation insurance coverage also has the potential to reduce tobacco-related population disparities.[6,14,17,37] Comprehensive cessation coverage can also support providers in their efforts to offer patients effective cessation treatments.[14,17] Finally, health systems cessation interventions can increase patients' use of available coverage.[14,17]

One important function of state tobacco control programs is to educate key stakeholders—including private and public health care systems, health insurers, the state Medicaid program, and employers—on the meaning of comprehensive cessation coverage and the importance and benefits of implementing such coverage. Educating employers on these topics is important because employers can play a key role in expanding cessation coverage by demanding such coverage and because self-insured employers are in a position to directly provide such coverage.[14,17]

For cessation insurance coverage to be effective in increasing cessation, it is important for it to be comprehensive in scope. Comprehensive coverage includes all evidence-based cessation treatments—including individual, group, and telephone counseling—and all seven Food and Drug Administration (FDA) approved cessation medications (bupropion, varenicline, and five forms of nicotine replacement therapy (NRT), including the patch, gum, lozenge, inhaler, and nasal spray). Comprehensive cessation coverage also eliminates or minimizes cost sharing and other barriers to accessing this coverage.[38] Finally, comprehensive cessation coverage includes proactively promoting the coverage to ensure that smokers and their health care providers are aware of it, thus increasing the chances that they will use it, and documenting and reporting utilization of the coverage.[14,38-41]

In January 2011, the Office of Personnel Management (OPM) implemented a cessation benefit for federal employees through the Federal Employees Health Benefits Program.[42] Highlights of that benefit, which is a model of comprehensive, evidence-based coverage, are listed in the following box.

Components of the Cessation Benefit Available to Federal Employees through the Federal Employees Health Benefits Program[42]

- Individual, group, and telephone counseling.
- All seven FDA-approved cessation medications, including both prescription and over-the-counter medications.
- Coverage for two quit attempts per year, with four counseling sessions per attempt.
- No copays, coinsurance, or deductibles.
- No annual or lifetime limits.

Once comprehensive cessation coverage has been achieved, state tobacco control programs may want to consider working with private and public health care systems, health insurers, employers, and other partners to publicize this coverage to smokers and their health care providers and to monitor its utilization.[39–41] High utilization is essential for a cessation benefit to be effective, because even the most comprehensive cessation coverage will have little impact if smokers and providers are not aware of it or don't use it.[39–41] In assessing the quality of cessation coverage, it is important to take into account barriers to access and utilization, as well as the cessation treatments covered.

In addition to working with the state Medicaid program to expand Medicaid cessation coverage, state programs can also seek to expand cessation coverage for state employees.[37] These employees typically make up a significant proportion of the state workforce, and the cessation coverage offered to this group can serve as a model for private employers and health plans.[37] Another approach taken by several states is to mandate private health insurers to provide some level of cessation coverage.[37]

Results of Massachusetts' Medicaid Cessation Benefit Implemented in 2006

- The benefit was utilized by about 37% of Medicaid recipients who smoked, or more than 70,000 individuals in its first 2½ years.[43]
- The smoking rate among Medicaid enrollees fell from 38.3% to 28.3%.[43]
- Annual hospital admissions for heart attacks and other acute heart disease diagnoses among Medicaid enrollees who used the benefit fell by 46% and 49%, respectively.[44]
- The benefit was found to generate a return on investment of $3.12 in cost savings from averted hospitalizations for acute cardiovascular events for every dollar spent on it.[45]

Several provisions in the Affordable Care Act expand private and Medicaid cessation coverage.[9,37,46] The legislation requires non-grandfathered private plans to cover, with no cost-sharing, preventive services that receive an 'A' or 'B' rating from the U.S. Preventive Services Task Force, which includes tobacco cessation treatments.[9,37,46] This requirement also applies to the insurance plans available to the individual and small group health insurance markets through each state's Health Insurance Marketplace.[9,37] Neither the Task Force recommendations nor the U.S. Department of Health and Human Services rules implementing the relevant provisions of the Act clearly define the specifics of the required tobacco cessation coverage; thus, these specifics remain somewhat open to interpretation.[37,47,48] To the extent possible, it is important for state tobacco control programs to work with large health insurers to ensure that they realize the full potential of these provisions by implementing comprehensive, evidence-based cessation coverage.

As of October 2010, the Affordable Care Act requires state Medicaid programs to cover cessation counseling for pregnant women.[9,37,46] Effective January 2014, the legislation bars these programs from excluding FDA-approved cessation medications from their coverage for all Medicaid enrollees.[9,37,46] In addition, states that choose to expand Medicaid eligibility must provide tobacco cessation coverage to newly eligible adults through a benchmark benefit package.[9,37] State Medicaid programs are also eligible for an increased federal medical assistance percentage if they provide recommended clinical preventive services, including tobacco cessation treatment, to traditional Medicaid recipients without cost sharing.[9,46] State tobacco control programs can work with state Medicaid programs to ensure that the potential of these provisions is fully realized. Medicaid enrollees smoke at higher rates than the general population, and smoking-related diseases in this population are a major driver of increasing state and federal Medicaid costs.[37,49]

Another provision of the Affordable Care Act allows health insurers in the individual and small group markets to charge tobacco users higher premiums than nontobacco users, up to a ratio of 1.5 to 1.0.[9,37,46] States retain the ability to reduce the ratio or to prohibit this practice entirely,[9,37] and several states have reportedly done so.[37] Although imposing higher premiums on tobacco users could motivate them to quit, it could also lead them to misrepresent their tobacco use status, avoid seeking cessation assistance, or forego health insurance, and could impose a prohibitive cost burden on low-income tobacco users.[37,50] The rule implementing this provision seeks to avert such outcomes by requiring health insurers in the small group market to allow tobacco users the opportunity to avoid paying the full amount of the tobacco rating factor by participating in a wellness program.[51,52] It is important for state tobacco control programs to monitor the implementation of this provision, and states may choose to restrict or prohibit the practice of charging tobacco users higher premiums if negative effects become apparent.

Separate from the Affordable Care Act, the Centers for Medicare and Medicaid Services has in recent years taken several steps to expand cessation coverage for Medicare enrollees, who comprise another potentially vulnerable population.[37] This coverage now includes individual counseling and prescription cessation medications, but not comprehensive cessation coverage.[37] There are opportunities to promote Medicare cessation benefits to increase their utilization.[37]

Sample State Activities: Expanding Insurance Coverage of Proven Cessation Treatments

- Build and maintain a relationship with private health insurers, the state Medicaid program, the state employee health plan, and large employers and educate them about the definition of comprehensive cessation coverage and about the health and economic benefits of providing such coverage.

- Work with the state Medicaid program to ensure that both fee-for-service and managed-care Medicaid plans provide comprehensive cessation coverage.

- Promote and monitor utilization of the state Medicaid cessation benefit.

- Work with state government to ensure that state employees have comprehensive cessation coverage.

- Implement a state mandate requiring private health insurers to provide comprehensive cessation coverage.

- Monitor implementation and effects of the provisions of the Affordable Care Act that have the potential to expand cessation coverage, as well as the provision that allows health insurers to charge tobacco users higher premiums.

Supporting State Quitline Capacity

> Quitlines are telephone-based services that help tobacco users quit by providing callers with counseling, practical information on how to quit, referral to other cessation resources, and, in some states and for certain populations, FDA-approved cessation medications.[16] Quitlines potentially have broad reach, are effective with diverse populations, and increase quit rates.[14]
>
> State quitlines are one of the most accessible cessation resources and can efficiently reach large numbers of smokers.[14,16] In addition, quitlines are effective in reaching certain racial/ethnic populations, including African Americans, persons who predominantly speak Asian languages, and low-income smokers.[53-56]
>
> Quitlines are highly cost-effective relative to other commonly used disease prevention interventions.[14,57-59] State quitlines are also typically the most visible component of state cessation efforts and frequently serve as a hub or centerpiece of these efforts.[16] State quitlines can also serve as clearinghouses and referral/triage centers, educating callers about the cessation coverage available from their health insurer and referring callers to community cessation services.[1,16]
>
> State quitlines can play an important role in supporting and increasing provider cessation interventions by offering a resource for additional, more intensive cessation counseling.[20,60,61] Having the option of referring patients to state quitlines for follow-up assistance increases the likelihood that providers will intervene with patients who smoke.[20,60,61] Most state quitlines have established fax referral programs,[20] and many state quitlines are developing the capacity to accept e-referrals directly from patients' electronic health records and to electronically send patient reports to the referring provider/health care organization.

Notwithstanding their many advantages and potentially broad reach, state quitlines on average reach only about 1% of smokers annually.[62,63] This situation is largely a function of modest state funding for providing and promoting state quitline services.[62,63] Some states, employers, and health plans have attained quitline reach levels of 6% or more.[64,65] State quitlines should seek to reach 8% of their state's tobacco users annually, with a target of 90% of these callers accepting counseling services. These guidelines take into account the experiences of state quitlines that have achieved higher levels of reach for limited periods.[1,64,65] These guidelines are also based on expectations that more health care providers will refer patients to quitlines as a result of Meaningful Use and the adoption of electronic health records, that more health plans will refer their members to quitlines in response to the Affordable Care Act, and that CDC's National tobacco education campaigns will continue to drive more callers to 1-800-QUIT-NOW.

In developing funding and service models, it is crucial to balance reach and intensity. It is important for state quitlines to seek to ensure that all callers have access to a basic level of service while providing higher levels of service to certain populations that would otherwise lack access to such services. Ensuring that a basic level of quitline service is in place is important to support interventions that are likely to increase interest in quitting and calls to quitlines, such as national or state media campaigns and implementation of smokefree laws or tobacco price increases. State tobacco control programs can use several approaches to increase quitline reach, including paid media campaigns, promotion of cessation medicine giveaways, and outreach efforts to generate fax or electronic referrals from health care organizations and providers.[1,6,23,24,66,67]

It is also important for state tobacco control programs to consider the level of funding for quitline operations and promotion that can realistically be sustained over time and to explore long-term funding sources. For example, programs can establish public-private partnerships, in which health plans or employers reimburse the state quitline for services provided to their members/employees, or contract directly with a quitline vendor to provide these services.[67,68] The Colorado and Minnesota tobacco control programs worked with their states' major private health plans to implement the first and second models, respectively; both these partnerships have been successful and have remained in place for a number of years.[67,68] State tobacco control programs can also work with their state Medicaid programs to secure the 50% federal match for quitline counseling provided to

Medicaid enrollees, who typically account for a substantial proportion of state quitline callers.[69]

State quitlines should consider providing some form of cessation assistance to all callers, including ensuring that all callers who want to talk to a quitline coach receive at least one ten-minute reactive call (i.e., a call initiated by the caller in which brief counseling is offered). Beyond this initial call, state quitlines can offer an additional three proactive counseling calls (i.e., calls initiated by the quitline in which counseling is offered) to the uninsured and underinsured, persons enrolled in a plan through the state Health Insurance Marketplace, Medicaid enrollees, and members of health plans and employees of companies that have contracted with the state to receive quitline services. Callers with private health insurance that provides adequate cessation coverage can be directed to their insurer or employer for cessation services after receiving an initial counseling call, or alternatively, the cost of additional calls can be reimbursed by their insurer or employer.[67,68]

State quitlines can also provide a free 2-week starter supply of NRT patches or gum to: uninsured and underinsured callers, persons in state insurance marketplace plans, and Medicaid enrollees.[1] This can increase calls to the quitline from these populations and these callers' success rates.[6,66,70–72] Another priority activity is to conduct targeted outreach to increase the state quitline's reach to underserved populations with high smoking rates. Longer-term efforts include: developing the capacity to accept e-referrals from patient electronic health records; integrating telephone cessation services with text messaging interventions and cessation services provided through other technologies, such as the Web and social media; and re-engaging previous quitline callers who agree to be re-contacted in quit attempts.[6,73] Text messaging, Web, and social media interventions could potentially extend the reach and impact of quitlines, particularly among younger individuals.[14]

State quitlines may also consider revisiting their eligibility protocols and service offerings in light of changes in health insurance coverage resulting from the implementation of the Affordable Care Act, including changes in the proportion of adults covered by different types of health insurance and in the cessation coverage provided. For example, several studies have documented the beneficial impact of providing brief introductory courses of NRT through quitlines.[6,66,70–72] However, most of these studies were conducted at a time when over-the-counter NRT was not generally available as a covered medication through health insurance plans. Accordingly, it is important for state tobacco control programs to monitor the situation in their states as it evolves and to consider limiting state quitlines' provision of longer (e.g., 8 week) courses of NRT to the uninsured, as appropriate. State quitlines can also revise the information they provide on NRT on the basis of recent FDA changes to the warnings on labeling of over-the-counter NRT products regarding long-term use and combined use with other NRT products or cigarettes.[74]

Section A: Cessation Interventions — **Best Practices for Comprehensive Tobacco Control Programs**

Sample State Activities: Supporting State Quitline Capacity

- Ensure that all callers receive some form of cessation assistance and that all callers who want to talk to a quitline coach receive at least one 10-minute reactive call.

- Ensure that all uninsured and underinsured callers and callers enrolled in state insurance marketplaces and Medicaid are offered three proactive counseling calls in addition to the reactive call and a free 2-week starter supply of NRT patches or gum.

- Ensure that all members of health plans and employees of companies that have contracted with the state quitline to receive quitline services are offered three proactive counseling calls in addition to the reactive call and a free 2-week starter supply of NRT patches or gum.

- Establish public-private partnerships under which health plans and employers either reimburse the state quitline for services provided to their members/employees or provide their own quitline services to these groups.

- Secure the federal Medicaid quitline match.

- Conduct targeted outreach to increase the state quitline's reach to underserved populations with high smoking rates, including promoting the national Spanish-language quitline portal 1-855-DÉJELO-YA (1-855-335-3569) and the national Asian-language quitline.

- Develop the capacity to accept e-referrals from patient electronic health records.

- Integrate quitline services with text messaging by referring callers to NCI's text messaging program.

- Re-engage previous quitline callers who agree to be re-contacted in quit attempts.

Achieving Equity to Eliminate Tobacco-Related Disparities

Significant population disparities exist with regard to tobacco cessation.[12,14] For example, recent data suggest that African American adults are more likely to express interest in quitting and more likely to have tried to quit in the past year than white adults, but are less likely to use proven treatments and are less likely to succeed in quitting.[12] Similarly, adults of lower socio-economic status express significant interest in quitting, but are more likely to be uninsured or on Medicaid and are less likely to receive cessation assistance.[14] Medicaid enrollees smoke at higher rates than the general population[37,49] and also express similar interest in quitting smoking as smokers with private insurance but are less likely to succeed.[12] One likely reason for this population's lower quit rates is that few state Medicaid programs provide comprehensive coverage of cessation treatments.[37]

Adults with mental illness have a much higher smoking prevalence than adults without mental illness, smoke more cigarettes per month, and are less likely to quit smoking.[14,75] Potential reasons that smokers with mental illness are less likely to quit include higher levels of nicotine addiction among this population and less access to cessation treatment, which may result from a lack of financial resources, a lack of health insurance, or a general reluctance of mental health care providers and facilities to address tobacco use in their patients.[14,75]

Lower quit rates in certain populations may result in part from environments and social norms that are less supportive of cessation and more supportive of tobacco use.[1,6,76,77] For example, blue collar and service workers have traditionally been less likely to be protected by smokefree workplace policies than white collar workers, and African Americans are less likely to live under smokefree home rules and are more likely to be exposed to secondhand smoke at work.[7,78,79] Similarly, until recently, many mental illness and substance abuse treatment facilities have not implemented tobacco-free or smokefree policies.[75] Comprehensive smokefree policies have been shown to effectively reduce population-level smoking, irrespective of socioeconomic status or race/ethnicity.[80] Because environments that are smokefree and norms that reduce the social acceptability of smoking motivate smokers to quit and make it easier for them to do so,[7,76,77] the lack of such environments and norms poses a barrier to cessation. State tobacco control programs can also increase cessation among population subgroups that make fewer quit attempts or are less likely to quit successfully by ensuring that settings where they spend time are smokefree. For example, state programs can seek to ensure that comprehensive state and local smokefree policies are fully implemented in all workplaces, and can work with primary and behavioral health care organizations serving these populations to implement tobacco-free campus policies.

In jurisdictions where comprehensive smokefree policies have already been implemented, other efforts can be made to encourage cessation, including the establishment of smokefree private settings, such as multiunit housing and vehicles; and tobacco price increases which motivate smokers to quit, and which low-income populations are especially responsive to. Increasing tax rates on tobacco products and dedicating a portion of the resulting revenue to fund cessation services for low-income populations can be an effective way to increase cessation in these populations.[6,81]

As illustrated in some of the examples cited above, lower quit rates in certain populations are often driven in part by reduced access to and use of evidence-based cessation treatments, which in turn results in less success in quitting.[12,14] One important way to improve cessation outcomes in populations with lower quit rates is to provide these populations with comprehensive cessation coverage.[6,14,37] Reducing barriers to accessing proven cessation treatments, including language and cost barriers, would be expected to increase quit attempts, use of effective cessation treatments, and success in quitting in these populations.[6,14,37] Providing comprehensive state Medicaid coverage would have a substantial impact, and is one of the most important steps a state can take to increase cessation and reduce tobacco use.[37,43–45]

Another effective approach is to conduct outreach and education to ensure that health care organizations serving these vulnerable populations with high smoking rates, such as federally qualified health centers, mental health care facilities, and substance abuse treatment facilities, integrate tobacco dependence treatment into routine health care delivery. Additionally, state tobacco control programs can address population disparities by conducting targeted outreach to increase the state quitline's reach to underserved populations with high smoking rates. This can include promoting national quitline resources developed to assist these populations, such as the national Spanish-language quitline portal 1-855-DÉJELO-YA (1-855-335-3569) and the national Asian-language quitline.

Budget

Promoting Health Systems Change/Expanding Cessation Insurance Coverage

The tobacco control goal of health systems change is to increase health care providers' identification of and intervention with patients who smoke. Because more than 80% of smokers see a physician each year, the clinical setting is an important channel for motivating smokers to quit and for delivering evidence-based cessation treatments. In addition, as noted previously, by removing barriers to accessing effective cessation treatments, expanding cessation insurance coverage increases the number of smokers who attempt to quit, who use effective treatments, and who successfully quit. As a result, it is important for state tobacco control programs to work with health systems as part of a comprehensive approach to encourage and help smokers to quit.

The budget recommendation for the state program for this component includes $150,000 per state, in addition to $17,850,000 allocated across states in proportion to total population, for grants to selected health care organizations, health insurers, and employers to evaluate cessation interventions, document the results, including cost-effectiveness and return on investment, and develop and disseminate reports on the findings.

Efforts to promote health systems change and expand cessation insurance coverage are demanding and time-intensive, requiring a sophisticated understanding of tobacco cessation and health care systems and sustained relationship-building with health care organizations, health insurers, and the state Medicaid program. Therefore, it is important to ensure that the tobacco control program's staff includes a dedicated, full-time cessation coordinator to oversee its cessation efforts, as well as additional staff and/or contractual personnel to conduct academic detailing and outreach to health care systems and insurers and to conduct data collection and analysis around cessation interventions and outcomes, including examining data from electronic health records and claims data.

Supporting State Quitline Capacity

The goal of state quitlines is to provide a convenient, readily accessible, evidence-based cessation service for smokers who want help quitting, a referral option for health care organizations and providers, and a clearinghouse for other cessation resources. Budget recommendations for this component are based on the percent of a state's smokers calling the state quitline (or other quitlines that health plans or employers have contracted with) for assistance each year, with a lower bound of 8% (*minimum* level) and an upper bound of 13% (*recommended* level). These parameters are based on the level of reach recommended in *Best Practices—2007*, combined with the updated assumption that 90% of callers will accept counseling and NRT.

These budget recommendations are based on offering all callers a single 10-minute reactive call and offering callers who are uninsured, underinsured, or enrolled in state insurance marketplaces or Medicaid three additional proactive counseling calls. The recommendations assume that callers who accept counseling will be provided with a total of four calls at a cost of $45.60 per call and that callers who accept medication will be provided with 2 weeks of NRT patches or gum at a cost of $38.00 per caller, with these estimates being based on state experience. In order to support population-based interventions such as smokefree policies and mass-media campaigns, state tobacco control programs may want to consider covering the cost of providing the initial reactive call during periods when such interventions are being implemented. During periods when such interventions are not being implemented, state quitlines can shift the cost of the initial call to other payers, except for uninsured and underinsured callers and callers enrolled in insurance through the state marketplaces and Medicaid.

It is assumed that the state program will cover 100% of the cost of providing the three proactive counseling calls to uninsured callers, underinsured callers, and callers who are enrolled in state insurance marketplaces and 50% of the cost of providing counseling to Medicaid callers, on the basis of the state quitline securing the 50% federal match for quitline counseling provided to Medicaid enrollees. In addition, it is assumed that the state tobacco control program will cover 100% of the cost of providing 2 weeks of NRT (patches or gum) to callers who are uninsured, underinsured, or enrolled in insurance through state marketplaces or Medicaid. Finally, it is assumed that other callers will have the costs of the three proactive quitline counseling calls and the 2 weeks of NRT borne by their payers. The payer will vary depending on the callers' insurance coverage, the quitline they call, and whether the state quitline has developed public-private partnerships with health plans and/or employers and secured the federal match for quitline counseling provided to Medicaid enrollees.

Providing Cessation Services Via Other Technologies

Emerging technologies, such as text messaging, Web, and social media interventions, could potentially extend the reach and increase the impact of quitlines by complementing telephone cessation assistance with quitting motivation and support delivered through other modalities.[14] These interventions are in some ways more convenient and readily accessible than quitlines and might engage young adult smokers, who may be especially likely to use these technologies and may prefer receiving cessation support through these familiar channels.[6,14] Budget recommendations for this component of the report are based on a fixed cost of $135,000 per state. Because these communication channels may continue to evolve and expand over time, it is important for state tobacco control programs to annually assess whether it may be cost-effective to increase this funding level to meet their goals.

References

1. Centers for Disease Control and Prevention. *Best Practices for Comprehensive Tobacco Control Programs — 2007.* Atlanta: U.S. Department of Health and Human Services, Centers for Disease Control and Prevention, National Center for Chronic Disease Prevention and Health Promotion, Office on Smoking and Health, 2007.

2. U.S. Department of Health and Human Services. Reducing Tobacco Use: *A Report of the Surgeon General.* Atlanta: U.S. Department of Health and Human Services, Centers for Disease Control and Prevention, National Center for Chronic Disease Prevention and Health Promotion, Office on Smoking and Health, 2000.

3. Institute of Medicine. *Ending the Tobacco Problem: A Blueprint for the Nation.* Washington: The National Academies Press, 2007.

4. U.S. Department of Health and Human Services. *The Health Consequences of Smoking: A Report of the Surgeon General.* Atlanta: U.S. Department of Health and Human Services, Centers for Disease Control and Prevention, National Center for Chronic Disease Prevention and Health Promotion, Office on Smoking and Health, 2004.

5. Jha P, Ramasundarahettige C, Landsman V, Rostron B, Thun M, Anderson RN, McAfee T, Peto R. 21st-century hazards of smoking and benefits of cessation in the United States. *New England Journal of Medicine* 2013;368(4):341–50.

6. The Guide to Community Preventive Services. Reducing tobacco use and secondhand smoke exposure; <http://www.thecommunityguide.org/tobacco/index.html>; accessed: December 2, 2013.

7. U.S. Department of Health and Human Services. *The Health Consequences of Involuntary Exposure to Tobacco Smoke: A Report of the Surgeon General.* Atlanta: U.S. Department of Health and Human Services, Centers for Disease Control and Prevention, Coordinating Center for Health Promotion, National Center for Chronic Disease Prevention and Health Promotion, Office on Smoking and Health, 2006.

8. Rigotti NA. Integrating comprehensive tobacco treatment into the evolving US health care system. *Archives of Internal Medicine* 2011;171(1):53–5.

9. *Patient Protection and Affordable Care Act,* Public Law 111-148, U.S. Statutes at Large 119 (2010):124.

10. Holahan J, Buettgens M, Carroll C, Dorn S. The Cost and Coverage Implications of the ACA Medicaid Expansion: National and State-by-State Analysis. Washington: The Urban Institute, 2012.

11. Zhu SH, Lee M, Zhuang YL, Gamst A, Wolfson T. Interventions to increase smoking cessation at the population level: how much progress has been made in the last two decades? Tobacco Control 2012;21(2):110–8.

12. Centers for Disease Control and Prevention. Quitting smoking among adults — United States, 2001–2010. *Morbidity and Mortality Weekly Report* 2011;60(44):1513–9.

13. Shiffman S, Brockwell SE, Pillitteri JL, Gitchell JG. Use of smoking-cessation treatments in the United States. *American Journal of Preventive Medicine* 2008;34(2):102–11.

14. Fiore MC, Jaen CR, Baker TB, et al. *Treating Tobacco Use and Dependence: 2008 Update.* Clinical Practice Guideline. Rockville, MD: U.S. Department of Health and Human Services, Public Health Service, 2008.

15. Ossip-Klein DJ, Giovino GA, Megahed N, Black PM, Emont SL, Stiggins J, Shulman E, Moore L. Effects of a smoker's hotline: results of a 10-county self-help trial. *Journal of Consulting and Clinical Psychology* 1991;59(2):325–32.

16. Centers for Disease Control and Prevention. *Telephone Quitlines: A Resource for Development, Implementation, and Evaluation.* Atlanta: U.S. Department of Health and Human Services, Centers for Disease Control and Prevention, National Center for Chronic Disease Prevention and Health Promotion, Office on Smoking and Health, 2004.

17. Fiore MC, Keller PA, Curry SJ. Health systems changes to facilitate the delivery of tobacco-dependence treatment. *American Journal of Preventive Medicine* 2007;33(6 Suppl):349S–356S.

18. Centers for Disease Control and Prevention. National Health Interview Survey; <http://www.cdc.gov/nchs/nhis.htm>; accessed: December 2, 2013.

19. Land TG, Rigotti NA, Levy DE, Schilling T, Warner D, Li W. The effect of systematic clinical interventions with cigarette smokers on quit status and the rates of smoking-related primary care office visits. *PLoS ONE* 2012;7(7):e41649.

20. Warner DD, Land TG, Rodgers AB, Keithly L. Integrating tobacco cessation quitlines into health care: Massachusetts, 2002–2011. *Preventing Chronic Disease* 2012;9:110343.

21. Schauer GL, Thompson JR, Zbikowski SM. Results from an outreach program for health systems change in tobacco cessation. *Health Promotion Practice* 2012;13(5):657–65.

22. Redmond LA, Adsit R, Kobinsky KH, Theobald W, Fiore MC. A decade of experience promoting the clinical treatment of tobacco dependence in Wisconsin. *Wisconsin Medical Journal* 2010;109(2):71–8.

23. Sheffer MA, Baker TB, Fraser DL, Adsit RT, McAfee TA, Fiore MC. Fax referrals, academic detailing, and tobacco quitline use: a randomized trial. *American Journal of Preventive Medicine* 2012; 42(1):21–8.

24. Bernstein SL, Jearld S, Prasad D, Bax P, Bauer U. Rapid implementation of a smokers' quitline fax referral service in an urban area. *Journal of Health Care for the Poor and Underserved* 2009;20(1):55–63.

25. Katz DA, Holman J, Johnson S, Hillis SL, Ono S, Stewart K, et al. Implementing smoking cessation guidelines for hospitalized veterans: effects on nurse attitudes and performance. *Journal of General Internal Medicine* 2013;28(11):1420–9.

26. Katz DA, Holman JE, Nugent AS, Baker LJ, Johnson SR, Hillis SL, et al. The emergency department action in smoking cessation (EDASC) trial: impact on cessation outcomes. *Nicotine & Tobacco Research* 2013;15(6):1032–43.

27. Kisuule F, Necochea A, Howe EE, Wright S. Utilizing audit and feedback to improve hospitalists' performance in tobacco dependence counseling. *Nicotine & Tobacco Research* 2010;12(8):797–800.

28. Centers for Medicare and Medicaid Services. Meaningful Use; <http://www.cms.gov/Regulations-and-Guidance/Legislation/EHRIncentivePrograms/Meaningful_Use.html>; accessed: December 2, 2013.

29. Boyle R, Solberg L, Fiore M. Use of electronic health records to support smoking cessation. *Cochrane Database of Systematic Reviews* 2011, Issue 12. Art. No.: CD008743. DOI: 10.1002/14651858.CD008743.pub2.

30. Bentz CJ, Bayley KB, Bonin KE, Fleming L, Hollis JF, Hunt JS, LeBlanc B, McAfee T, Payne N, Siemienczuk J. Provider feedback to improve 5A's tobacco cessation in primary care: a cluster randomized clinical trial. *Nicotine & Tobacco Research* 2007;9(3):341–9.

31. Linder JA, Rigotti NA, Schneider LI, Kelley JHK, Brawarsky P, Haas JS. An electronic health record–based intervention to improve tobacco treatment in primary care: a cluster-randomized controlled trial. *Archives of Internal Medicine* 2009;169(8):781–7.

32. Greenwood DA, Parise CA, MacAller TA, Hankins AI, Harms KR, Pratt LS, Olveda JE, Buss KA. Utilizing clinical support staff and electronic health records to increase tobacco use documentation and referrals to a state quitline. *Journal of Vascular Nursing* 2012;30(4):107–11.

33. Lindholm C, Adsit R, Bain P, Reber PM, Brein T, Redmond L, Smith, SS, and Fiore MC. A demonstration project for using the electronic health record to identify and treat tobacco users. *Wisconsin Medical Journal* 2010;109(6):335–40.

34. The Joint Commission. Core Measure Sets: Tobacco Treatment; <http://www.jointcommission.org/core_measure_sets.aspx>; accessed: December 2, 2013.

35. Fiore MC, Goplerud E, Schroder SA. The Joint Commission's new tobacco-cessation measures — will hospitals do the right thing? *New England Journal of Medicine* 2012;366(13):1172–4.

36. Partnership for Prevention. *Helping Patients Quit: Implementing the Joint Commission Tobacco Measure Set in Your Hospital.* Washington: Partnership for Prevention, 2011. <http://www.prevent.org/Publications-and-Resources.aspx/hpq_full_final_10-31-11.pdf>; accessed: December 2, 2013.

37. American Lung Association. *Helping Smokers Quit: Tobacco Cessation Coverage 2012.* Washington: American Lung Association, 2012. <http://www.lung.org/assets/documents/publications/smoking-cessation/helping-smokers-quit-2012.pdf>; accessed: December 2, 2013.

38. Centers for Disease Control and Prevention. Coverage for Tobacco Use Cessation Treatments; <http://www.cdc.gov/tobacco/quit_smoking/cessation/coverage/index.htm>; accessed: December 2, 2013.

39. McMenamin SB, Halpin HA, Ibrahim JK, Orleans CT. Physician and enrollee knowledge of Medicaid coverage for tobacco dependence treatments. *American Journal of Preventive Medicine* 2004;26(2):99–104.

40. McMenamin SB, Halpin HA, Bellows NM. Knowledge of Medicaid coverage and effectiveness of smoking treatments. *American Journal of Preventive Medicine* 2006;31(5):369–74.

41. Keller PA, Christiansen B, Kim SY, Piper ME, Redmond L, Adsit R, Fiore MC. Increasing consumer demand among Medicaid enrollees for tobacco dependence treatment: the Wisconsin "Medicaid covers it" campaign. *American Journal of Health Promotion* 2011;25(6):392–5.

42. U.S. Office of Personnel Management. Special Initiatives: Quit Smoking; <http://www.opm.gov/healthcare-insurance/special-initiatives/quit-smoking/>; accessed: December 2, 2013.

43. Land T, Warner D, Paskowsky M, Cammaerts A, Wetherell L, Kaufmann R, Zhang L, Malarcher A, Pechacek T, Keithly L. Medicaid coverage for tobacco dependence treatments in Massachusetts and associated decreases in smoking prevalence. *PLoS ONE* 2010;5(3):e9770.

44. Land T, Rigotti NA, Levy DE, Paskowsky M, Warner D, Kwass JA, Wetherell L, Keithly L. A longitudinal study of Medicaid coverage for tobacco dependence treatments in Massachusetts and associated decreases in hospitalizations for cardiovascular disease. *PLoS Med* 2010;7(12):e1000375.

45. Richard P, West K, Ku L. The return on investment of a Medicaid tobacco cessation program in Massachusetts. *PLoS ONE* 2012;7(1):e29665.

46. University of Wisconsin Center for Tobacco Research and Intervention (UW-CTRI). Summary of Selected Tobacco, Prevention, and Public Health Provisions from H.R. 3590, the Patient Protection and Affordable Care Act, and H.R. 4872, the Health Care and Education Reconciliation Act of 2010, Signed into Law March 23, 2010 and March 30, 2010 respectively. University of Wisconsin Center for Tobacco Research and Intervention, 2010; <http://www.ctri.wisc.edu/HC.Providers/reform/aca/hcrtobacco2010.pdf>; accessed: December 2, 2012.

47. Kofman M, Dunton K, Senkewicz MB. Implementation of Tobacco Cessation Coverage under the Affordable Care Act: Understanding how Private Health Insurance Policies Cover Tobacco Cessation Treatments. Washington: Georgetown University Health Policy Institute, 2012; <http://www.tobaccofreekids.org/pressoffice/2012/georgetown/coveragereport.pdf>; accessed: December 2, 2013.

48. Centers for Disease Control and Prevention. Health plan implementation of U.S. Preventive Services Task Force A and B recommendations — Colorado, 2010. *Morbidity and Mortality Weekly Report* 2011;60(39):1348–50.

49. Armour BS, Finkelstein EA, Fiebelkorn IC. State-level Medicaid expenditures attributable to smoking. *Preventing Chronic Disease* 2009;6(3):A84.

50. Curtis R, Neuschler E. Tobacco Rating Issues and Options for California under the ACA. Washington: Institute for Health Policy Solutions, 2012; <http://www.ihps.org/pubs/Tobacco_Rating_Issue_Brief_21June2012.pdf>; accessed: December 2, 2013.

51. *Federal Register*. Patient Protection and Affordable Care Act; Health Insurance Market Rules; Rate Review; < https://www.federalregister.gov/articles/2013/02/27/2013-04335/patient-protection-and-affordable-care-act-health-insurance-market-rules-rate-review >; accessed: December 2, 2013.

52. *Federal Register*. Incentives for Nondiscriminatory Wellness Programs in Group Health Plans; < https://www.federalregister.gov/articles/2013/06/03/2013-12916/incentives-for-nondiscriminatory-wellness-programs-in-group-health-plans >; accessed: December 2, 2013.

53. Zhu SH, Gardiner P, Cummins S, Anderson C, Wong S, Cowling D, Gamst A. Quitline utilization rates of African-American and white smokers: the California experience. *American Journal of Health Promotion* 2011;25(5 Suppl):51S–58S.

54. Rabius V, Wiatrek D, McAlister AL. African American participation and success in telephone counseling for smoking cessation. *Nicotine & Tobacco Research* 2012;14(2):240–2.

55. Zhu SH, Wong S, Stevens C, Nakashima D, Gamst A. Use of smokers' quitline by Asian language speakers: results from 15 years of operation in California. *Research and Practice* 2010;100(5):846–52.

56. Miller CL, Sedivy V. Using a quitline plus low-cost nicotine replacement therapy to help disadvantaged smokers to quit. *Tobacco Control* 2009;18(2):144–9.

57. Hollis JF, McAfee TA, Fellows JL, et al. The effectiveness and cost effectiveness of telephone counseling and the nicotine patch in a state tobacco quitline. *Tobacco Control* 2007;16(Suppl 1):i53–i59.

58. Lal A, Mihalopoulos C, Wallace A, et al. The cost-effectiveness of call-back counselling for smoking cessation. *Tobacco Control* Published Online First: June 8, 2013. DOI: 10.1136/tobaccocontrol-2012-050907.

59. Tomson T, Helgason AR, Gilljam H. Quitline in smoking cessation: a cost-effectiveness analysis. International *Journal of Technology Assessment in Health Care* 2004;20(4):469–74.

60. Rothemich SF, Woolf SH, Johnson RE, Devers KJ, Flores SK, Villars P, Rabius V, McAfee T. Promoting primary

Section A: Cessation Interventions

care smoking cessation support with quitlines: the QuitLink Randomized Controlled Trial. *American Journal of Preventive Medicine* 2010;38(4):367–74.

61. Shelley D, Cantrell J. The effect of linking community health centers to a state-level smoker's quitline on rates of cessation assistance. *BMC Health Services Research* 2010;10:25. DOI: 10.1186/1472-6963-10-25.

62. Anderson CM, Zhu SH. Tobacco quitlines: looking back and looking ahead. *Tobacco Control* 2007;16(Suppl 1):i81–i86.

63. Keller PA, Feltracco A, Bailey LA, Li Z, Niederdeppe J, Baker T, Fiore MC. Changes in tobacco quitlines in the United States, 2005–2006. *Preventing Chronic Disease* 2010;7(2):A36.

64. Woods SS, Haskins AE. Increasing reach of quitline services in a US state with comprehensive tobacco treatment. *Tobacco Control* 2007;16(Suppl 1):i33–i36.

65. National Jewish Medical and Research Center. Tobacco Cessation Outcome Results for the State Tobacco Educational and Prevention Partnership (STEPP) — August 2007. Denver, CO: National Jewish Medical and Research Center, 2007.

66. Bush TM, McAfee T, Deprey M, Mahoney L, Fellows JL, McClure J, Cushing C. Impact of a free nicotine patch starter kit on quit rates in state quitline. *Nicotine & Tobacco Research* 2008;10(9):1511–6.

67. Schillo BA, Wendling A, Saul J, Luxenberg MG, Lachter R, Christenson M, An LC. Expanding access to nicotine replacement therapy through Minnesota's QUITLINE partnership. *Tobacco Control* 2007;16(Suppl 1):i37–i41.

68. Partnership for Prevention. *Colorado Tobacco Cessation and Sustainability Partnership: A Case Study: A Collaborative Approach to Meeting the U.S. Preventive Services Task Force Recommendations on Tobacco Cessation Screening and Intervention.* Washington: Partnership for Prevention, 2011.

69. Centers for Medicare and Medicaid Services. State Medicaid Director Letter on New Medicaid Tobacco Cessation Services, June 24, 2011; <http://www.cms.gov/smdl/downloads/SMD11-007.pdf>; accessed: December 2, 2013.

70. An LC, Schillo BA, Kavanaugh AM, Lachter RB, Luxenberg MG, Wendling AH, Joseph AM. Increased reach and effectiveness of a statewide tobacco quitline after the addition of access to free nicotine replacement therapy. *Tobacco Control* 2006;15(4):286–93.

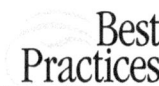

71. Cummings KM, Fix B, Celestino P, Carlin-Menter S, O'Connor R, Hyland A. Reach, efficacy, and cost-effectiveness of free nicotine medication giveaway programs. *Journal of Public Health Management Practice* 2006;12(1):37–43.

72. Campbell SL, Lee L, Haugland C, Helgerson SD, Harwell TS. Tobacco quitline use: enhancing benefit and increasing abstinence. *American Journal of Preventive Medicine* 2008;35(4):386–8.

73. National Cancer Institute. Smokefree TXT; <http://www.smokefree.gov/smokefreetxt/default.aspx>; accessed: December 2, 2013.

74. *Federal Register*. U.S. Department of Health and Human Services, Food and Drug Administration. Modifications to labeling of nicotine replacement therapy products for over-the-counter human use. Docket No. FDA-2013-N-0341. Fed. Reg. 2013;78(63):19718–21.

75. Centers for Disease Control and Prevention. Vital Signs: Current cigarette smoking among adults aged ≥ 18 years with mental illness — United States, 2009–2011. *Morbidity and Mortality Weekly Report* 2013;62(05):81–7.

76. Hopkins DP, Razi S, Leeks KD, Kaira GP, Chattopadhyay SK, Soler RE, the Task Force on Community Preventive Services. Smokefree policies to reduce tobacco use: a systematic review. *American Journal of Preventive Medicine* 2010;38(2 Suppl):275S–289S.

77. Zhang X, Cowling DW, Tang H. The impact of social norm change strategies on smokers' quitting behaviours. *Tobacco Control* 2010;19(Suppl 1):i51–i55.

78. Arheart KL, Lee DJ, Dietz NA, Wilkinson JD, Clark III JD, LeBlanc WG, Serdar B, Fleming LE. Declining trends in serum cotinine levels in US worker groups: the power of policy. *Journal of Occupational and Environmental Medicine* 2008;50(1):57–63

79. King BA, Dube SR, Homa DM. Smoke-free rules and secondhand smoke exposure in homes and vehicles among US adults, 2009–2010. *Preventing Chronic Disease* 2013;10:120218.

80. Dinno A, Glantz S. Tobacco control policies are egalitarian: a vulnerabilities perspective on clean indoor air laws, cigarette prices, and tobacco use disparities. *Social Science and Medicine* 2009;68(8):1439–47.

81. International Agency for Research on Cancer (IARC). IARC Handbooks of Cancer Prevention, Tobacco Control, Vol. 14: *Effectiveness of Tax and Price Policies for Tobacco Control*. Lyon, France: IARC, 2011.

IV. Surveillance and Evaluation

Justification

Publicly financed programs need to have accountability and demonstrate effectiveness, as well as have access to timely data that can be used for program improvement and decision making. Therefore, a critical infrastructure component of any comprehensive tobacco control program is a surveillance and evaluation system that can monitor and document key short-term, intermediate, and long-term outcomes within populations.[1,2] Data obtained from surveillance and evaluation systems can be used to inform program and policy direction, demonstrate program effectiveness, ensure accountability to those with fiscal oversight, and engage stakeholders.[2-6]

Surveillance and evaluation planning may be integrated into the overall strategic plan of a comprehensive tobacco control program and be compatible and comparable with systems in other states and nationally.[2] A strategic plan, with well-defined goals, objectives, and outcomes, requires appropriate data collection methods that can monitor the program, as well as evaluate key outcome indicators in a valid manner.[7]

Additionally, the collection of baseline data related to each objective and outcome indicator is critical to ensuring that program-related effects can be clearly measured.[3,5] For this reason, surveillance and evaluation systems must have priority in the strategic planning process.

Surveillance

Surveillance is the process of continuously monitoring attitudes, behaviors, and health outcomes over time.[8] Although data gathered by surveillance systems can be useful for evaluation, they serve other purposes besides evaluation. For example, data collection for the purposes of evaluation is more flexible than for surveillance and may allow program areas to be assessed in greater depth. Statewide tobacco control surveillance programs should consider monitoring the achievement of the four overarching goals of comprehensive tobacco control programs:

- Preventing initiation among youth and young adults
- Promoting quitting among adults and youth
- Eliminating exposure to secondhand smoke
- Identifying and eliminating tobacco-related disparities among population groups

Implementing state surveillance systems, such as the Behavioral Risk Factor Surveillance System (BRFSS), Youth Risk Behavior Surveillance System (YRBSS), Pregnancy Risk Assessment Monitoring System (PRAMS), and the Adult or Youth Tobacco Surveys (ATS, YTS), affords each state the opportunity to collect data on tobacco use behaviors and other important risk factors and health outcomes.[9-11] Data from these systems also allow a state to compare its individual program impact and long-term tobacco indicators with other states as well as with national benchmarks from national surveillance systems. In addition to the standard core questions included in these surveys, there is flexibility to add state-specific questions and modules. States also have the flexibility to increase sample size in order to capture local and specific population data or to provide more data on intermediate performance outcomes.

Evaluation

Evaluation has been defined as the systematic collection of information about the activities, characteristics, and results of programs to make judgments about the program, improve or further develop program effectiveness, inform decisions about future programming, and/or increase understanding.[12] Evaluation data can be used for assessing the effectiveness of individual program activities, program improvement, decision making, and to engage stakeholders. However, in order to do all these things, a written evaluation plan must first be integrated with the overall strategic plan. An effective evaluation plan:[13]

- Is collaboratively developed with a stakeholder workgroup
- Is responsive to program changes and priorities
- Covers multiple years if projects are ongoing

- Addresses the entire program rather than focusing on a single funding source, objective, or activity

States can also consider publishing their evaluation results in order to contribute to the scientific literature on best practices for tobacco control programs.[7]

A typical approach to evaluation in public health is to design data-collection systems that monitor progress toward meeting a program's process and outcome objectives.[8] Process evaluations are used to document how well a program has been implemented and are conducted periodically during a program.[8] This type of an evaluation is used to examine the program's operations, including which activities are taking place, who is conducting the activities, and who is reached through the activities. In contrast, outcome evaluations are used to assess the effectiveness of a program on the stated short-term, intermediate, and long-term objectives.[8] This type of evaluation assesses what has occurred because of the program and whether the program has achieved its objectives.

The program's stages of development must be considered in the evaluation plan, particularly when determining the appropriate evaluation questions. Outcome evaluations are best conducted only when the program is mature enough to produce the intended outcome. However, consideration for future evaluations can be included in the evaluation plan so that programs can prepare datasets and baseline information for evaluations that consider more distal impacts and outcomes.[14]

An evaluation plan can include both process and outcome evaluation questions at the same time.[14] Program evaluation also requires that a wide range of short-term, intermediate, and long-term indicators of program effectiveness be measured, including changes in policies, social norms, and exposure of individuals and communities to statewide and local program efforts. For example, evaluation efforts might include countermarketing surveillance to track new products and examine the impact of pro-tobacco influences, including tobacco product marketing, pricing, and promotion. Additional indicators for program evaluation can include, but need not be limited to, vital statistics, quitline utilization, policy compliance and enforcement, air quality, or media related measures. Practice-based criteria to be considered in the selection of indicators for monitoring and evaluation have previously been listed elsewhere.[15]

Qualities of Effective Program Evaluations[2,13,16]

- Ongoing and include a written evaluation plan that is integrated with the program's overall strategic plan.

- Flexible, adaptive, transparent, and designed to inform and engage stakeholders at each step, including implementation, interpretation, dissemination, and utilization of results.

- Focus on priority evaluation questions and not special research interests or what is easiest to implement.

- Confirm that the methods align with the evaluation questions and objectives.

- Identify credible evidence and verify its accuracy and appropriateness with stakeholders.

- Make effective use of surveillance data by linking statewide and local program efforts to monitor progress toward program objectives.

- Plan for dissemination and sharing of lessons learned throughout the evaluation process.

- Include technical assistance to disseminate information on how to implement effective evaluations to funded sites, partners, stakeholders, and local programs.

Selected Surveillance and Evaluation Resources

Surveillance and evaluation can be conducted simultaneously.[8] To assess tobacco-use prevention and control efforts adequately, states will usually need to supplement surveillance data with data collected to answer specific evaluation questions. States can collect data on, for example, knowledge, attitudes, behaviors, and environmental indicators. They can also collect information on infrastructure, program planning, and implementation to document and measure the effectiveness of a program, including its policy and media efforts. Some existing tools for both surveillance and evaluation at the state and national levels include:

Adult Tobacco Survey (ATS): ATS is a state level landline and cellular telephone survey of adults aged 18 years or older.[17] Core questions assess adults' knowledge, attitudes, and behaviors related to tobacco use, secondhand smoke exposure, use of cessation assistance, and their awareness of and support for evidence-based policy interventions.

In addition to these core questions, ATS allows for the inclusion of questions addressing state-specific program activities. CDC's *Key Outcome Indicators for Evaluating Comprehensive Tobacco Control Programs* was used to inform the development of the ATS survey.[1] CDC's Office on Smoking and Health can provide technical assistance to states regarding the administration of ATS.

Behavioral Risk Factor Surveillance System (BRFSS): BRFSS is a state-based telephone survey of non-institutionalized U.S. adults aged 18 years or older that CDC initiated in 1984.[9] Data are currently collected annually in all 50 states, the District of Columbia, and five U.S. territories. With assistance from CDC, state health departments contract with telephone call centers to conduct BRFSS surveys continuously throughout the year using a standardized core questionnaire and optional modules plus additional state-added questions. Beginning in 2011, several enhancements were made to BRFSS to ensure optimal survey coverage and validity, including the addition of cellular telephone households and improvements to the sampling methods and statistical weighting.[18]

National Adult Tobacco Survey (NATS): NATS is a landline and cellular phone survey of U.S. adults aged 18 years or older.[19] NATS was first conducted during 2009–2010, and the sample was designed to provide data representative at both national and state levels.[19] Additional waves of NATS were fielded in 2012-2013 and 2013-2014 in collaboration with FDA; however state-level estimates will only be obtainable during 2009-2010.

National Youth Tobacco Survey (NYTS): NYTS is a nationally representative school-based survey of youth in middle school (grades 6–8) and high school (9–12).[20] NYTS cannot be used to obtain state-level estimates, but estimates from the survey can serve as a national benchmark for those obtained from state YTS surveys. NYTS is a multitopic survey that includes measures that assess tobacco use, cessation, knowledge and attitudes, access, media and advertising, and secondhand smoke exposure.[1] Survey years include 2000, 2002, 2004, 2006, 2009, 2011, and 2012. As of 2012, NYTS will be fielded annually until 2017 in collaboration with FDA.

Pregnancy Risk Assessment Monitoring System (PRAMS): PRAMS is a surveillance system that CDC and state health departments have conducted in multiple phases since 1987; PRAMS data were most recently collected in 2011.[11] PRAMS collects state-specific, population-based data on maternal attitudes and experiences before, during, and shortly after pregnancy. The PRAMS questionnaire comprises two parts, including core questions that are asked by all states and a pretested list of standard questions that CDC or individual states develop. The core PRAMS questionnaire includes questions on maternal tobacco consumption.

Quitline Minimum Data Set (MDS): The quitline MDS identifies a recommended set of indicators to assist in assessing telephone quitline performance, improving the quality of telephone quitlines, identifying knowledge gaps, and designing new strategies to fill the identified gaps.[21]

State Tobacco Activities Tracking and Evaluation (STATE) System: The STATE System is an online data warehouse that includes epidemiologic data on many long-term key outcome indicators, as well as economic data and tobacco-related state legislation.[22]

Tobacco Use Supplement to the Current Population Survey (TUS-CPS): TUS-CPS is an in-person and telephone survey of U.S. adults aged 18 years and older that was administered during 1992–1993, 1995–1996, 1998–1999, 2002–2003,

Section A: Surveillance and Evaluation ——————————————————— for **Comprehensive Tobacco Control Programs**

2006–2007, and 2010–2011; the next wave is slated for 2014–2015.[23] These tobacco-use modules provide national and state-specific estimates on factors such as tobacco use, quit attempts, secondhand smoke exposure, smokefree policies, and clinician cessation counseling.

Youth Risk Behavior Surveillance System (YRBSS): YRBSS is a national school-based survey of middle and high school students conducted annually by CDC.[10] YRBSS also includes state, territorial, tribal, and local surveys conducted by state, territorial, and local education and health agencies and tribal governments. YRBSS monitors six types of health-risk behaviors that contribute to leading causes of death and disability among youth and adults, including tobacco use.

Youth Tobacco Survey (YTS): YTS is a school-based, state-level survey of students in grades 6–12.[24] Core questions assess students' knowledge, attitudes, and behaviors related to tobacco use and exposure to secondhand smoke, as well as their exposure to prevention curricula, community programs, and media messages aimed at preventing and reducing youth tobacco use. In addition to the core set of questions, YTS allows for the inclusion of questions addressing state-specific program activities. CDC's *Key Outcome Indicators for Evaluating Comprehensive Tobacco Control Programs* was used to inform the development of the YTS survey.[1] CDC's Office on Smoking and Health can provide technical assistance to states regarding the administration of YTS.

In addition to the previously described surveillance and evaluation tools, several resources are available to provide guidance and support to states on the selection and implementation of appropriate surveillance and evaluation data systems.

Surveillance and Evaluation Resources

- *Surveillance and Data Resources for Comprehensive Tobacco Control Programs* provides a summary of tobacco-related measures, sampling frames, and methodology for multiple national and state surveys as well as tools for use in conducting surveillance and evaluation efforts.[25]

- *Introduction to Program Evaluation for Comprehensive Tobacco Control Programs* is a "how-to" guide for planning and implementing evaluation activities.[8]

- *Key Outcomes Indicators for Evaluating Comprehensive Tobacco Control Programs* provides information on selecting evidence-based indicators and linking them to program outcomes.[1]

- *Introduction to Process Evaluation in Tobacco Use Prevention and Control* provides guidance to states on how to evaluate inputs, activities, and outputs of a tobacco control logic model.[26]

- *Developing an Effective Evaluation Plan* can help public health program managers, administrators, and evaluators develop an effective evaluation plan in the context of the planning process. It is intended to be used along with other evaluation resources and is not a complete resource on how to implement program evaluation.[13] For example, disseminating surveillance and evaluation findings in brief updates or newsletters to key stakeholders may also be beneficial.

- *Developing an Effective Evaluation Report* can help public health program managers, administrators, and evaluators develop an effective evaluation report. It is intended to be used along with other evaluation resources and is not a complete resource on how to write reports or communicate and use your evaluation results.[14]

- *Impact and Value: Telling Your Program's Story* offers public health program managers practical steps for creating success stories that highlight their achievements.[27]

State-Level Examples

Surveillance and evaluation data can be used by states in multiple ways to help inform and sustain comprehensive state tobacco control programs. For example, states can collect their own state-level surveillance and evaluation data using previously developed instruments and resources, supplement existing surveillance systems with indicators related to specific state tobacco control program objectives, or utilize secondary data sources to assess key indicators and make comparisons with other states or national benchmarks. Examples of some recent state-level surveillance and evaluation activities are described below.

The New York Tobacco Control Program has fielded variations of the ATS and YTS questionnaires regularly for more than a decade. The program utilizes these data to provide a comprehensive summary of multiple key outcomes indicators in its annual *Independent Evaluation Report*.[28] These reports help to clearly and objectively illustrate the impact that the state tobacco control program has had on key outcome indicators, as well as to highlight gaps that need to be addressed in the future.

Multiple states supplement the core BRFSS questionnaire with optional modules to inform state-level tobacco control program efforts.[9] For example, in 2011, two optional modules pertaining to smoking cessation and secondhand smoke were proposed and ratified. The smoking cessation module was administered by Arizona, Guam, Kentucky, Louisiana, Maryland, and Nebraska; the secondhand smoke module was administered by Guam, Indiana, Kentucky, Louisiana, and Mississippi.

The Public Health Division of the Wyoming Department of Health recently utilized state-level data from the 2009–2010 NATS to measure progress toward attaining the objectives of Wyoming's Tobacco Prevention and Control Program. A summary of the findings were described in a comprehensive report organized according to CDC's four overarching goals for comprehensive tobacco control programs.[7,29]

Achieving Equity to Eliminate Tobacco-Related Disparities

Dissemination of surveillance and evaluation data that show disparities can be very effective in mobilizing community involvement. In order to develop effective interventions and monitor progress, most states need more information on populations disproportionately affected by tobacco use.[7] Many of the surveillance and evaluation resources described in this report include questions related to population characteristics for which tobacco-related disparities have been shown to exist, including but not limited to: race/ethnicity, educational attainment, income, occupation, geographic location, sex, age, sexual orientation and gender identity, veteran and military status, disability status, mental health status, and substance abuse conditions.

However, it is important to note that existing surveillance and evaluation methods may not provide adequate sample size or enough information to fully characterize health disparities related to tobacco use. Therefore, additional data collection systems or approaches may be needed. For example, the use of oversampling, combining multiple years of data, and qualitative methods are often necessary to adequately assess these outcomes among some population groups.

Budget

All federally funded tobacco prevention and control programs are expected to engage in strategic surveillance and program evaluation activities. To accomplish this, best practices dictate that 10% of total annual tobacco control program funds be allocated for surveillance and evaluation.

It is important that tobacco control programs develop and maintain the appropriate infrastructure to enhance their surveillance and evaluation resources as needed. For example, conducting a detailed evaluation of a specific intervention, such as a cohort study to assess the effectiveness of a media campaign, can be resource intensive.[7,30] Similarly, additional resources beyond the standard 10% of tobacco control program funds may also be required for developing increased technical capacity of local programs to perform process and outcome evaluation.[7,30] For example, in California, every grantee was required to spend 10% of its budget on evaluating its own activities. To aid this activity, the state program published a directory of evaluation consultants and funded a local program evaluation center that provides technical assistance to contractors.[31]

In addition, programs may need to be flexible in shifting funding to address new and emerging products or trends of public health concern. For example, recent increases in electronic cigarette marketing and use warrant targeted surveillance, monitoring, and evaluation that may not have been recognized if a program's plan was developed several years ago.

Realizing the national goal of eliminating tobacco-related disparities will require improved collection and use of standardized data to correctly identify disparities in both health outcomes and interventional efficacy.[7] Accordingly, additional resources may also be required to fund data collection mechanisms and standardized systems to better characterize health disparities related to tobacco use among special populations and to effectively measure progress.

References

1. Starr G, Rogers T, Schooley M, Porter S, Wiesen E, Jamison N. *Key Outcome Indicators for Evaluating Comprehensive Tobacco Control Programs*. Atlanta: Centers for Disease Control and Prevention, National Center for Chronic Disease Prevention and Health Promotion, Office on Smoking and Health, 2005.

2. Lavinghouze R, Snyder K. Developing your evaluation plans: a critical component of public health program infrastructure. *American Journal of Health Education* 2013;44(4):237–43.

3. Giovino GA, Biener L, Hartman AM, Marcus SE, Schooley MW, Pechacek TF, Vallone D. Monitoring the tobacco use epidemic. I. Overview: optimizing measurement to facilitate change. *Preventive Medicine* 2009;48(1 Suppl):4S–10S.

4. Institute of Medicine. *Ending the Tobacco Problem: A Blueprint for the Nation*. Washington: National Academies Press, 2007.

5. World Health Organization (WHO). *WHO Report on the Global Tobacco Epidemic, 2008: The MPOWER Package*. Geneva, Switzerland: WHO, 2008.

6. Lavinghouze R, Snyder K, Rieker P, Ottoson J. Consideration of an applied model of public health program infrastructure. *Journal of Public Health Management and Practice* 2013;19(6):E28–E37. DOI: 10.1097/PHH.0b013e31828554c8.

7. Centers for Disease Control and Prevention. *Best Practices for Comprehensive Tobacco Control Programs — October 2007*. Atlanta: U.S. Department of Health and Human Services, Centers for Disease Control and Prevention, National Center for Chronic Disease Prevention and Health Promotion, Office on Smoking and Health, 2007.

8. MacDonald G, Starr G, Schooley M, Yee SL, Klimowski K, Turner K. *Introduction to Program Evaluation for Comprehensive Tobacco Control Programs*. Atlanta: Centers for Disease Control and Prevention, National Center for Chronic Disease Prevention and Health Promotion, Office on Smoking and Health, 2001.

9. Centers for Disease Control and Prevention. Behavioral Risk Factor Surveillance System; <http://www.cdc.gov/brfss/>; accessed: December 2, 2013.

10. Centers for Disease Control and Prevention. Youth Risk Behavior Surveillance System; <http://www.cdc.gov/HealthyYouth/yrbs/index.htm>; accessed: December 2, 2013.

11. Centers for Disease Control and Prevention. Pregnancy Risk Assessment Monitoring System; <http://www.cdc.gov/PRAMS/>; accessed: December 2, 2013.

12. Patton, MQ. *Utilization-Focused Evaluation*. 4th ed. Los Angeles: Sage Publications, 2008.

13. Centers for Disease Control and Prevention. *Developing an Effective Evaluation Plan*. Atlanta: U.S. Department of Health and Human Services, Centers for Disease Control and Prevention, National Center for Chronic Disease Prevention and Health Promotion, Office on Smoking and Health, Division of Nutrition, Physical Activity, and Obesity, 2011.

14. Centers for Disease Control and Prevention. *Developing an Effective Evaluation Report*. Atlanta: Centers for Disease Control and Prevention, National Center for Chronic Disease Prevention and Health Promotion, Office on Smoking and Health, Division of Nutrition, Physical Activity and Obesity, 2013.

15. MacDonald, G. Criteria for Selection of High-Performing Indicators: A Checklist to Inform Monitoring and Evaluation; <http://www.wmich.edu/evalctr/checklists/>; accessed: December 2, 2013.

16. Lavinghouze SR, Price AW, Smith KA. The program success story: a valuable tool for program evaluation. *Health Promotion Practice* 2007;8(4):323–31.

17. McClave AK, Whitney N, Thorne SL, Mariolis P, Dube SR, Engstrom M. Adult Tobacco Survey — 19 states, 2003–2007. *Morbidity and Mortality Weekly Report Surveillance Summary* 2010;59(SS3):1–75.

18. Centers for Disease Control and Prevention. Methodologic changes in the Behavioral Risk Factor Surveillance System in 2011 and potential effects on prevalence estimates. *Morbidity and Mortality Weekly Report* 2012;61(22):410–3.

19. King BA, Dube SR, Tynan MA. Current tobacco use among adults in the United States: findings from the National Adult Tobacco Survey. *American Journal of Public Health* 2012;102(11):e93–e100.

20. Centers for Disease Control and Prevention. National Youth Tobacco Survey; <http://www.cdc.gov/tobacco/data_statistics/surveys/nyts/>; accessed: December 2, 2013.

21. North American Quitline Consortium. Quitline Minimal Data Set; <http://www.naquitline.org/?page=mds>; accessed: December 2, 2013.

22. Centers for Disease Control and Prevention. State Tobacco Activities Tracking and Evaluation

(STATE) System; <http://www.cdc.gov/tobacco/statesystem>; accessed: December 2, 2013.

23. National Cancer Institute. Tobacco Use Supplement to the Current Population Survey; <http://riskfactor.cancer.gov/studies/tus-cps/>; accessed: December 2, 2013.

24. Centers for Disease Control and Prevention. Youth Tobacco Survey; <http://www.cdc.gov/tobacco/data_statistics/surveys/YTS/index.htm>; accessed: December 2, 2013.

25. Yee SL, Schooley M. *Surveillance and Evaluation Data Resources for Comprehensive Tobacco Control Programs*. Atlanta: Centers for Disease Control and Prevention, National Center for Chronic Disease Prevention and Health Promotion, Office on Smoking and Health, 2001.

26. Centers for Disease Control and Prevention. *Introduction to Process Evaluation in Tobacco Use Prevention and Control*. Atlanta: U.S. Department of Health and Human Services, Centers for Disease Control and Prevention, National Center for Chronic Disease Prevention and Health Promotion, Office on Smoking and Health, 2008.

27. Centers for Disease Control and Prevention. *Impact and Value: Telling Your Program's Story*. Atlanta: Centers for Disease Control and Prevention, National Center for Chronic Disease Prevention and Health Promotion, Division of Oral Health, 2007.

28. New York State Department of Health. Reports, Brochures, and Fact Sheets; <http://www.health.ny.gov/prevention/tobacco_control/reports_brochures_fact-sheets.htm>; accessed: December 2, 2013.

29. Wyoming Survey and Analytic Center. 2010 Wyoming National Adult Tobacco Survey Report; < http://wysac1.uwyo.edu/wysac/ReportView.aspx?DocId=529&A=1>; accessed: December 2, 2013.

30. World Health Organization European Working Group on Health Promotion Evaluation. *Health Promotion Evaluation: Recommendations to Policy-makers: Report of the WHO European Working Group on Health Promotion Evaluation*. Copenhagen, Denmark: World Health Organization, Regional Office for Europe, 1998.

31. Roeseler A, Hagaman T, Kurtz C. The use of training and technical assistance to drive and improve performance of California's Tobacco Control Program. *Health Promotion and Practice* 2011;12(6 Suppl 2):130S–143S.

V. Infrastructure, Administration, and Management

Justification

A comprehensive tobacco control program requires considerable funding to implement; therefore, a fully functioning infrastructure must be in place in order to achieve the capacity to implement effective interventions.[1-6] Sufficient capacity is essential for program sustainability, efficacy, and efficiency, and enables programs to plan their strategic efforts, provide strong leadership, and foster collaboration among the state and local tobacco control communities. An adequate number of skilled staff is also necessary to provide or facilitate program oversight, technical assistance, and training.

Staff resources dedicated to administration and management of infrastructure development and maintenance activities include:[1]

- Engaging in strategic planning to guide program efforts and resources to accomplish their goals

- Recruiting and developing qualified and diverse technical, program, and administrative staff

- Awarding and monitoring program contracts and grants, coordinating implementation across program areas, and assessing grantee program performance

- Developing and maintaining a real-time fiscal management system

- Increasing capacity at the local level by providing ongoing training and technical assistance

- Coordinating across chronic disease programs and with local coalitions and partners

- Educating the public and decision makers on the health effects of tobacco and effective, evidence-based program and policy interventions

In part due to rising fiscal challenges, an increasing number of state health departments have taken steps to combine efforts and increase efficiency by realigning disease-specific programs into a coordinated chronic disease infrastructure. These steps often include developing and implementing cross-cutting policies, conducting integrated chronic disease surveillance and evaluation, targeting interventions toward areas of the state with the greatest burden, and developing coordinated messaging to reach people with comorbidities.

Addressing tobacco control strategies in the broader context of chronic diseases can be beneficial from the standpoint of enhanced coordination and efficiencies related to basic administrative functions, as well as the potential to synergistically increase the reach and efficacy of interventions.

However, the realignment of disease-specific programs may also result in the dismantling of dedicated staff and resources for state tobacco control programs. Potential strategies to reduce any adverse impact of infrastructural changes on state tobacco control programs include:

- Establishing or maintaining a full-time tobacco control program manager

- Retaining core staff positions necessary and unique to tobacco control interventions

- Developing and sustaining collaborations with external partners

- Expanding staff and partner capacity through trainings for state and community staff

- Exploring alternative funding opportunities to support staffing for a broad chronic disease infrastructure that includes a highly functioning tobacco control program

Functioning Infrastructure

Program infrastructure is the foundation that supports program capacity, implementation, and sustainability.[2-7] The Component Model of Infrastructure (CMI) defines infrastructure in a practical, actionable, and evaluable manner so that grant planners, evaluators, and program implementers can link infrastructure to capacity, measure success, and increase the likelihood for sustainable health achievements (See Figure 2). According to CMI, functioning program infrastructure includes five core components: networked partnerships, multilevel leadership, engaged data, managed resources, and responsive plans/planning.[2-5]

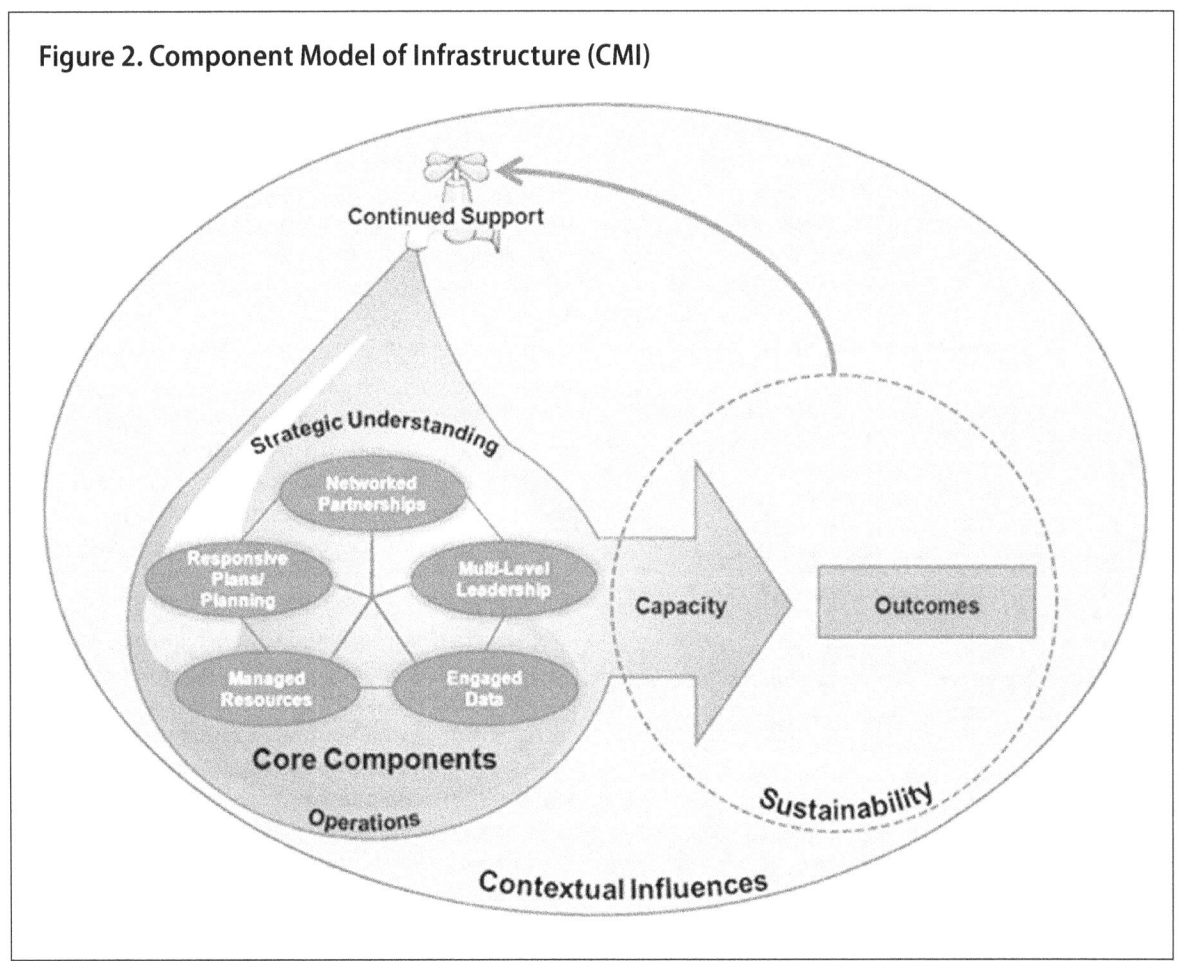

Figure 2. Component Model of Infrastructure (CMI)

Networked Partnerships: Strategic collaboration is crucial at the national, state, and local levels. These partnerships can be made between multiple types of organizations and content areas to promote progress toward health goals. Although many partners are working towards a common mission, they may fill different roles. In this way, networked partnerships can work to ensure the accomplishment of all activities necessary to achieve public health goals.

Multi-level Leadership: Leaders and champions can be identified and nurtured at all levels. This includes leadership above the tobacco control program in the health department or other organizational unit where the program is located; leadership within the program beyond the program manager; leadership among partners and other chronic disease areas; and leadership in local programs. Leadership at all levels is necessary to develop relationships and to ensure functioning program infrastructure and progress toward health goals.

Engaged Data: Data can be used in a manner that engages staff, partners, decision makers, and local programs to act. Data should not merely be collected and displayed but also used to promote public health goals. Therefore, training, technical assistance, and follow-through are necessary to ensure the proper utilization of data.

Managed Resources: A functional infrastructure requires resources beyond financing, including an adequate number of staff and partners who are qualified and have diverse technical, program, and administrative skills. Staff, partners, and local programs must also have the necessary training and skills to effectively implement the tobacco control program.

Responsive Plans/Planning: Responsive strategic plans are dynamic and evolve in response to contextual influences, such as changes in scientific evidence, priorities, funding levels, and external support. In addition, the planning process is collaborative and includes viewpoints from multiple stakeholders.[8] This process fosters shared ownership and responsibility for the goals and objectives between the state program, partners, and local programs.

Multiple states have successfully realized the core components of the CMI. For example, Oregon has three levels of *Networked Partnerships*, including local community partners, chronic disease areas, and other agencies such as substance abuse and mental health treatment facilities. In 2011, networked partnerships were instrumental in successfully producing Oregon's first-ever report on how managed care organizations serving Medicaid clients identify tobacco users and provide tobacco cessation services, and determine whether those services met evidence-based standards.

Similarly, Utah utilized *Multi-level Leadership* to address cessation via a project addressing the health burden of tobacco use among those suffering from substance abuse or mental health issues. The program developed a leadership team for the project that included leaders from the substance abuse and mental health programs, as well as local health departments, non-profits, clinical directors, and clients. They worked with every leader to ensure that each felt ownership of the project.

For *Engaged Data*, New York developed a surveillance and evaluation system using program logic models that included evaluation data from locally funded programs. Data have been used to evaluate the state's comprehensive smokefree law using multiple indicators, including hospitality venue sales, indoor air quality, biomarkers of secondhand smoke exposure in employees, and long term measures such as hospital admissions for heart attacks.

For *Managed Resources*, Massachusetts adheres to a model in which core capabilities are kept in house and the rest are outsourced. This model includes cross-training and preparing staff to move into leadership roles, as well as maintaining a robust training program that ensures staff and partners' capabilities grow and keep pace with technological advancement.

Finally, for *Responsive Plans/Planning*, Colorado created a flexible, budget- and evidence-based, strategic plan that enabled their staff to respond to changes, including funding reductions. Key components of the plan comprised evaluation as well as infrastructure development and maintenance, which included training and technical assistance.

However, CMI goes beyond the core components in its depiction of functioning program infrastructure. The five core components of the CMI model are enveloped in contextual influences as well as supporting components,

Section A: Infrastructure, Administration, and Management — for **Comprehensive Tobacco Control Programs**

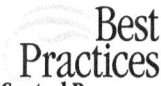

including *Strategic Understanding* and *Operations*.[2–7] This type of framework enables a tobacco control program to quickly align with strategic plans and partners, irrespective of what opportunities or challenges emerge.

The *Strategic Understanding* component encompasses the ideas, guidelines, and thinking that initiate, nurture, and sustain infrastructure. Core concepts include perception of the problem as a public health issue—both among the public and decision makers—as well as planning for program sustainability at the beginning rather than at the end of a funding cycle. A sustainability plan can be one of the critical plans included under the *Responsive Plans/Planning* component, along with the strategic plan.

The *Operations* component comprises the day-to-day work structures, communications, and procedures associated with implementing a comprehensive tobacco control program. Operations can include roles and responsibilities of staff, partners, and local programs, as well as a formal and effective communications system. This communication system needs to include methods for communicating data, evaluation results, program operations, funding guidelines, and goals and objectives, not only among staff, but also within the health department, across connected programs and chronic disease areas, and with partners, local programs, and decision makers.

Capacity

Capacity is the ability to implement evidence-based interventions.[2–4] Once infrastructure is built and properly supported, it facilitates the capacity to take advantage of opportunities, create opportunities, and to defend against threats to the achievement of the program goals. Building and maintaining the infrastructure to support capacity to provide guidance, technical assistance, and coordination among programs and partners are critical, foundational activities for comprehensive tobacco control programs.[1–4,9,10]

State experience has shown the importance of having all of the program's components coordinated and working together. Program management and coordination present a challenge in that a comprehensive program involves multiple state agencies (e.g. public health, education, and law enforcement) and levels of local government, other public health programs, and numerous health-related voluntary organizations, coalitions, and community groups.

Administration and management staff provide the stable foundation on which any program is built and maintained. Accordingly, an adequate number of skilled staff is required to fully implement and sustain a comprehensive tobacco control program. The exact percentage of full time equivalent positions required will depend on the state population, current tobacco control progress, and program needs. However, all programs should consider having staff to cover the necessary components of a comprehensive tobacco control program.

Ideal Staffing Plan for a Comprehensive Tobacco Control Program

- Program director.
- Policy coordinator.
- Communications specialist.
- Cessation coordinator.
- Surveillance and evaluation staff.
- Fiscal management systems staff.
- Administrative staff.

Continued Support

Once a strong, functioning program infrastructure is in place, the cumulative effect of funding on program effectiveness becomes evident. Research shows that the longer states invest in comprehensive tobacco control programs, the greater and quicker the impact.[11–13] Because a significant amount of time and resources may be required to establish a functional infrastructure capable of implementing effective tobacco control interventions, it is critical to maintain that infrastructure.

CMI depicts the critical nature of continued support and the cyclical nature of maintaining functioning program infrastructure and its impact on outcomes and sustainability. Sustainability has been defined as the "existence of structures and processes that allow a program to leverage resources to effectively implement and maintain evidence-based policies and activities."[10] These structures and processes are embodied in the core and enveloping components of CMI.

Achieving Equity to Reduce Tobacco-Related Disparities

In order to adequately identify and effectively eliminate tobacco-related disparities, state tobacco control programs must implement a number of tobacco prevention and control strategies, including establishing infrastructure and building capacity.[14] These strategies help guide the development of policies and practices that reflect the principles of inclusion, cultural competency, and equity.

To support achieving equity and reaching the goal of identifying and eliminating tobacco-related disparities, it is crucial that state tobacco control programs work to achieve the infrastructure and capacity necessary to: conduct surveillance to identify populations disproportionately affected by tobacco use and disseminate the data; partner with population groups disproportionately affected by tobacco and the community organizations that serve them; ensure that disparity issues are an integral part of state and community tobacco control strategic plans, fund organizations that can effectively reach, involve, and mobilize these populations; and provide culturally competent technical assistance and training to grantees and partners.

This guidance highlights the minimum infrastructure and capacity needed by state tobacco control programs to pursue a strategic plan with initiatives that will most effectively achieve equity in tobacco prevention and control through the identification and elimination of tobacco-related disparities.

Budget

Best practices dictate that 5% of total annual tobacco control program funds be allocated for administration and management of infrastructure development and maintenance activities. This budget is for the administration and management of infrastructure, not for all infrastructure activities. This might include costs pertaining to office expenses, postage and shipping, printing and duplication, occupancy expenses, equipment and maintenance, training and travel, planning, coordination activities, as well as staff time directly related to core planning and program oversight functions.

Because of the importance of maintaining functioning infrastructure and the capacity to provide guidance, technical assistance, and coordination among programs and other key partners, the suggested target for administration and management of infrastructure activities should generally be 5% of a state's total CDC-recommended program budget, even if actual program funding is below the CDC-recommended level.

References

1. Centers for Disease Control and Prevention. *Best Practices for Comprehensive Tobacco Control Programs—October 2007.* Atlanta: U.S. Department of Health and Human Services, Centers for Disease Control and Prevention, National Center for Chronic Disease Prevention and Health Promotion, Office on Smoking and Health, 2007.

2. Lavinghouze SR, Snyder K, Rieker P, Ottsoson J. Consideration of an applied model of public health program infrastructure. *Journal of Public Health Management and Practice* 2013;19(6):E28–E37. DOI: 10.1097/PHH.0b013e31828554c8.

3. Lavinghouze SR. The difficulties and complexities of evaluating "inputs": the forgotten box of the logic model. Panel presentation #406 at the Twenty-Fifth Annual American Evaluation Association Conference; November 2011; Anaheim, CA.

4. Lavinghouze SR. The components of infrastructure: A model in progress. Panel presentation #576 at the Twenty-Fifth Annual American Evaluation Association Conference; November 2011; Anaheim, CA.

5. Lavinghouze, SR, Rieker P, Snyder K. The Component Model of Infrastructure (CMI): an infrastructure model for evaluating tobacco control programs. Evaluation ancillary meeting at the National Conference on Tobacco or Health; August 2012; Kansas City, MO.

6. Lavinghouze SR, Snyder K. Developing your evaluation plans: a critical component of public health program infrastructure. *American Journal of Health Education* 2013;44(4):237–43.

7. Centers for Disease Control and Prevention. *Developing an Effective Evaluation Report.* Atlanta: Centers for Disease Control and Prevention, National Center for Chronic Disease Prevention and Health Promotion, Office on Smoking and Health, Division of Nutrition, Physical Activity and Obesity, 2013.

8. Institute of Medicine. *Living Well with Chronic Illness: A Call for Public Health Action.* Washington: The National Academies Press, 2012.

9. Chapman R. Organization development in public health: A foundation for growth. 2010.

10. Schell SF, Luke DA, Schooley MW, Elliott MB, Herbers SH, Mueller NB, Bunger AC. Public health program capacity for sustainability: A new framework. *Implementation Science* 2013;8(15). DOI: 10.1186/1748-5908-8-15.

11. Farrelly MC, Pechacek TF, Chaloupka FJ. The impact of tobacco control program expenditures on aggregate cigarette sales: 1981–2000. *Journal of Health Economics* 2003;22(5):843–59.

12. Farrelly MC, Pechacek TF, Thomas KY, Nelson D. The impact of tobacco control programs on adult smoking. *American Journal of Public Health* 2008;98(2):304–9.

13. Farrelly MC, Loomis BR, Han B, Gfroerer J, Kuiper N, Couzens GL, Dube SR, Caraballo RS. A comprehensive examination of the influence of state tobacco control programs and policies on youth smoking. *American Journal of Public Health* 2013;103(3):549–55.

14. Fagan P, King G, Lawrence D, Petrucci SA, Robinson RG, Banks D, et al. Eliminating tobacco-related health disparities: directions for future research. *American Journal of Public Health* 2004;94(2):211–7.

Section B
Recommended Funding Levels for All 50 States and the District Of Columbia

Annual **Total Funding Levels** for State Programs

	Total Program Costs		State and Communication Interventions		Mass-Reach Health Communication Interventions	
	Minimum (millions)	Recommended (millions)	Minimum (millions)	Recommended (millions)	Minimum (millions)	Recommended (millions)
United States	**2,325.3**	**3,306.3**	**856.7**	**1,071.0**	**370.1**	**532.0**
Alabama	39.1	55.9	14.4	18.0	4.2	6.0
Alaska	7.5	10.2	3.3	4.1	1.0	1.4
Arizona	45.5	64.4	16.8	20.9	7.9	11.4
Arkansas	25.9	36.7	10.1	12.7	2.5	3.5
California	248.6	347.9	99.9	124.9	52.8	76.0
Colorado	37.4	52.9	13.2	16.4	6.9	9.9
Connecticut	22.7	32.0	9.1	11.4	2.6	3.7
Delaware	9.3	13.0	3.4	4.3	2.0	2.8
District of Columbia	7.8	10.7	3.4	4.2	1.4	2.0
Florida	135.5	194.2	44.9	56.2	25.9	37.2
Georgia	74.4	106.0	28.0	35.0	10.4	14.9
Hawaii	9.9	13.7	4.5	5.6	1.1	1.6
Idaho	11.3	15.6	4.7	5.8	1.5	2.1
Illinois	96.3	136.7	36.1	45.2	15.9	22.8
Indiana	51.2	73.5	18.8	23.5	5.1	7.3
Iowa	21.3	30.1	8.4	10.5	2.5	3.6
Kansas	19.8	27.9	8.4	10.5	1.3	1.9
Kentucky	39.2	56.4	15.2	19.0	2.4	3.5
Louisiana	41.8	59.6	15.6	19.5	5.7	8.1
Maine	11.2	15.9	4.1	5.2	1.6	2.3
Maryland	33.7	48.0	12.8	16.0	3.5	5.0
Massachusetts	47.0	66.9	16.9	21.2	8.9	12.8
Michigan	76.9	110.6	28.3	35.4	7.9	11.4
Minnesota	37.1	52.9	13.5	16.8	5.2	7.5
Mississippi	25.7	36.5	10.0	12.5	2.9	4.1
Missouri	50.7	72.9	17.4	21.8	7.5	10.8
Montana	10.5	14.6	4.0	5.0	2.2	3.1
Nebraska	14.7	20.8	5.3	6.6	2.5	3.6
Nevada	21.3	30.0	8.3	10.4	3.4	4.9
New Hampshire	11.7	16.5	4.0	5.0	2.8	4.1
New Jersey	72.7	103.3	23.4	29.2	19.1	27.5
New Mexico	16.3	22.8	7.4	9.3	1.3	1.8
New York	142.8	203.0	49.3	61.6	31.8	45.7
North Carolina	69.3	99.3	26.4	33.1	6.8	9.8
North Dakota	7.0	9.8	2.9	3.7	0.9	1.3
Ohio	92.0	132.0	34.3	42.9	10.0	14.4
Oklahoma	29.8	42.3	11.7	14.6	2.4	3.4
Oregon	27.7	39.3	10.3	12.9	4.1	5.9
Pennsylvania	97.3	140.0	32.7	40.8	14.8	21.3
Rhode Island	9.3	12.8	3.8	4.7	1.5	2.1
South Carolina	35.5	51.0	13.4	16.7	3.2	4.7
South Dakota	8.5	11.7	3.5	4.4	1.2	1.7
Tennessee	52.5	75.6	18.7	23.4	5.5	7.9
Texas	185.8	264.1	68.0	85.0	33.3	47.9
Utah	13.9	19.3	5.8	7.3	2.3	3.4
Vermont	6.1	8.4	2.5	3.1	1.1	1.6
Virginia	63.9	91.6	19.1	23.8	15.4	22.2
Washington	44.5	63.6	16.4	20.5	6.3	9.1
West Virginia	19.2	27.4	6.7	8.4	2.6	3.7
Wisconsin	40.0	57.5	14.7	18.4	4.4	6.4
Wyoming	6.2	8.5	2.9	3.6	0.6	0.9

Annual **Total Funding Levels** for State Programs

	Cessation Interventions		Surveillance and Evaluation		Infrastructure, Administration, and Management	
	Minimum (millions)	Recommended (millions)	Minimum (millions)	Recommended (millions)	Minimum (millions)	Recommended (millions)
United States	**795.1**	**1,271.9**	**202.6**	**287.7**	**100.8**	**143.7**
Alabama	15.4	24.6	3.4	4.9	1.7	2.4
Alaska	2.2	3.4	0.7	0.9	0.3	0.4
Arizona	14.8	23.7	4.0	5.6	2.0	2.8
Arkansas	9.9	15.7	2.3	3.2	1.1	1.6
California	63.5	101.6	21.6	30.3	10.8	15.1
Colorado	12.4	19.7	3.3	4.6	1.6	2.3
Connecticut	8.0	12.7	2.0	2.8	1.0	1.4
Delaware	2.7	4.2	0.8	1.1	0.4	0.6
District of Columbia	2.0	3.1	0.7	0.9	0.3	0.5
Florida	47.0	75.5	11.8	16.9	5.9	8.4
Georgia	26.3	42.3	6.5	9.2	3.2	4.6
Hawaii	3.0	4.7	0.9	1.2	0.4	0.6
Idaho	3.6	5.6	1.0	1.4	0.5	0.7
Illinois	31.7	50.9	8.4	11.9	4.2	5.9
Indiana	20.6	33.1	4.5	6.4	2.2	3.2
Iowa	7.6	12.1	1.9	2.6	0.9	1.3
Kansas	7.5	11.9	1.7	2.4	0.9	1.2
Kentucky	16.5	26.5	3.4	4.9	1.7	2.5
Louisiana	15.1	24.2	3.6	5.2	1.8	2.6
Maine	4.0	6.3	1.0	1.4	0.5	0.7
Maryland	13.0	20.7	2.9	4.2	1.5	2.1
Massachusetts	15.1	24.2	4.1	5.8	2.0	2.9
Michigan	30.7	49.4	6.7	9.6	3.3	4.8
Minnesota	13.6	21.7	3.2	4.6	1.6	2.3
Mississippi	9.5	15.1	2.2	3.2	1.1	1.6
Missouri	19.2	30.8	4.4	6.3	2.2	3.2
Montana	2.9	4.6	0.9	1.3	0.5	0.6
Nebraska	5.0	7.9	1.3	1.8	0.6	0.9
Nevada	6.8	10.8	1.9	2.6	0.9	1.3
New Hampshire	3.4	5.3	1.0	1.4	0.5	0.7
New Jersey	20.7	33.1	6.3	9.0	3.2	4.5
New Mexico	5.5	8.7	1.4	2.0	0.7	1.0
New York	43.1	69.2	12.4	17.7	6.2	8.8
North Carolina	27.1	43.5	6.0	8.6	3.0	4.3
North Dakota	2.3	3.5	0.6	0.9	0.3	0.4
Ohio	35.7	57.5	8.0	11.5	4.0	5.7
Oklahoma	11.8	18.8	2.6	3.7	1.3	1.8
Oregon	9.7	15.4	2.4	3.4	1.2	1.7
Pennsylvania	37.1	59.6	8.5	12.2	4.2	6.1
Rhode Island	2.8	4.3	0.8	1.1	0.4	0.6
South Carolina	14.3	23.0	3.1	4.4	1.5	2.2
South Dakota	2.7	4.1	0.7	1.0	0.4	0.5
Tennessee	21.4	34.4	4.6	6.6	2.3	3.3
Texas	60.2	96.7	16.2	23.0	8.1	11.5
Utah	4.0	6.1	1.2	1.7	0.6	0.8
Vermont	1.7	2.6	0.5	0.7	0.3	0.4
Virginia	21.0	33.6	5.6	8.0	2.8	4.0
Washington	16.0	25.7	3.9	5.5	1.9	2.8
West Virginia	7.4	11.7	1.7	2.4	0.8	1.2
Wisconsin	15.7	25.2	3.5	5.0	1.7	2.5
Wyoming	1.9	2.9	0.5	0.7	0.3	0.4

Annual **Per Capita Funding Levels** for State Programs

	Total Program Costs		State and Communication Interventions		Mass-Reach Health Communication Interventions	
	Minimum	Recommended	Minimum	Recommended	Minimum	Recommended
United States	**7.41**	**10.53**	**2.73**	**3.41**	**1.18**	**1.69**
Alabama	8.11	11.58	2.99	3.73	0.87	1.24
Alaska	10.22	14.00	4.51	5.61	1.37	1.91
Arizona	6.93	9.84	2.56	3.19	1.21	1.74
Arkansas	8.77	12.44	3.42	4.31	0.85	1.19
California	6.54	9.15	2.63	3.28	1.39	2.00
Colorado	7.20	10.20	2.54	3.16	1.33	1.91
Connecticut	6.30	8.92	2.53	3.18	0.72	1.03
Delaware	10.15	14.17	3.71	4.69	2.18	3.05
District of Columbia	12.37	16.91	5.38	6.64	2.21	3.16
Florida	7.00	10.07	2.32	2.91	1.34	1.93
Georgia	7.50	10.68	2.82	3.53	1.05	1.50
Hawaii	7.10	9.84	3.23	4.02	0.79	1.15
Idaho	7.08	9.73	2.95	3.63	0.94	1.32
Illinois	7.46	10.61	2.80	3.51	1.23	1.77
Indiana	7.83	11.24	2.88	3.59	0.78	1.12
Iowa	6.91	9.81	2.73	3.42	0.81	1.17
Kansas	6.86	9.68	2.91	3.64	0.45	0.66
Kentucky	8.96	12.87	3.47	4.34	0.55	0.80
Louisiana	9.10	12.95	3.39	4.24	1.24	1.76
Maine	8.38	11.94	3.08	3.91	1.20	1.73
Maryland	5.73	8.15	2.18	2.72	0.59	0.85
Massachusetts	7.08	10.08	2.54	3.19	1.34	1.93
Michigan	7.79	11.19	2.86	3.58	0.80	1.15
Minnesota	6.91	9.82	2.51	3.12	0.97	1.39
Mississippi	8.63	12.21	3.35	4.19	0.97	1.37
Missouri	8.43	12.10	2.89	3.62	1.25	1.79
Montana	10.42	14.52	3.98	4.97	2.19	3.08
Nebraska	7.94	11.23	2.86	3.56	1.35	1.94
Nevada	7.71	10.88	3.01	3.77	1.23	1.78
New Hampshire	8.88	12.54	3.03	3.79	2.12	3.10
New Jersey	8.20	11.64	2.64	3.29	2.15	3.10
New Mexico	7.83	10.91	3.55	4.46	0.62	0.86
New York	7.29	10.38	2.52	3.15	1.62	2.34
North Carolina	7.12	10.18	2.71	3.39	0.70	1.00
North Dakota	10.04	13.98	4.15	5.29	1.29	1.86
Ohio	7.97	11.45	2.97	3.72	0.87	1.25
Oklahoma	7.81	11.10	3.07	3.83	0.63	0.89
Oregon	7.11	10.09	2.64	3.31	1.05	1.51
Pennsylvania	7.62	10.97	2.56	3.20	1.16	1.67
Rhode Island	8.88	12.15	3.62	4.47	1.43	2.00
South Carolina	7.54	10.81	2.84	3.54	0.68	0.99
South Dakota	10.21	14.07	4.20	5.28	1.44	2.04
Tennessee	8.12	11.70	2.90	3.62	0.85	1.22
Texas	7.13	10.13	2.61	3.26	1.28	1.84
Utah	4.87	6.77	2.03	2.56	0.81	1.19
Vermont	9.74	13.41	3.99	4.95	1.76	2.56
Virginia	7.80	11.18	2.33	2.91	1.88	2.71
Washington	6.45	9.22	2.38	2.97	0.91	1.32
West Virginia	10.35	14.75	3.61	4.53	1.40	1.99
Wisconsin	6.99	10.04	2.57	3.21	0.77	1.12
Wyoming	10.78	14.76	5.03	6.25	1.04	1.56

Annual Per Capita Funding Levels for State Programs

	Cessation Interventions		Surveillance and Evaluation		Infrastructure, Administration, and Management	
	Minimum	Recommended	Minimum	Recommended	Minimum	Recommended
United States	**2.53**	**4.05**	**0.65**	**0.92**	**0.32**	**0.46**
Alabama	3.19	5.10	0.71	1.01	0.35	0.50
Alaska	3.01	4.65	0.89	1.22	0.44	0.61
Arizona	2.26	3.62	0.60	0.86	0.30	0.43
Arkansas	3.36	5.32	0.76	1.08	0.38	0.54
California	1.67	2.67	0.57	0.80	0.28	0.40
Colorado	2.39	3.80	0.63	0.89	0.31	0.44
Connecticut	2.23	3.54	0.55	0.78	0.27	0.39
Delaware	2.94	4.58	0.88	1.23	0.44	0.62
District of Columbia	3.16	4.90	1.08	1.47	0.54	0.74
Florida	2.43	3.91	0.61	0.88	0.30	0.44
Georgia	2.65	4.26	0.65	0.93	0.33	0.46
Hawaii	2.15	3.38	0.62	0.86	0.31	0.43
Idaho	2.26	3.51	0.62	0.85	0.31	0.42
Illinois	2.46	3.95	0.65	0.92	0.32	0.46
Indiana	3.15	5.06	0.68	0.98	0.34	0.49
Iowa	2.47	3.94	0.60	0.85	0.30	0.43
Kansas	2.60	4.12	0.60	0.84	0.30	0.42
Kentucky	3.77	6.05	0.78	1.12	0.39	0.56
Louisiana	3.28	5.26	0.79	1.13	0.40	0.56
Maine	3.01	4.74	0.73	1.04	0.36	0.52
Maryland	2.21	3.52	0.50	0.71	0.25	0.35
Massachusetts	2.27	3.64	0.62	0.88	0.31	0.44
Michigan	3.11	5.00	0.68	0.97	0.34	0.49
Minnesota	2.53	4.03	0.60	0.85	0.30	0.43
Mississippi	3.18	5.06	0.75	1.06	0.38	0.53
Missouri	3.19	5.11	0.73	1.05	0.37	0.53
Montana	2.89	4.58	0.91	1.26	0.45	0.63
Nebraska	2.69	4.26	0.69	0.98	0.35	0.49
Nevada	2.46	3.91	0.67	0.95	0.34	0.47
New Hampshire	2.57	4.01	0.77	1.09	0.39	0.55
New Jersey	2.34	3.73	0.71	1.01	0.36	0.51
New Mexico	2.64	4.17	0.68	0.95	0.34	0.47
New York	2.20	3.54	0.63	0.90	0.32	0.45
North Carolina	2.78	4.46	0.62	0.89	0.31	0.44
North Dakota	3.29	5.00	0.87	1.22	0.44	0.61
Ohio	3.09	4.98	0.69	1.00	0.35	0.50
Oklahoma	3.09	4.93	0.68	0.97	0.34	0.48
Oregon	2.49	3.95	0.62	0.88	0.31	0.44
Pennsylvania	2.91	4.67	0.66	0.95	0.33	0.48
Rhode Island	2.67	4.09	0.77	1.06	0.39	0.53
South Carolina	3.03	4.87	0.66	0.94	0.33	0.47
South Dakota	3.24	4.92	0.89	1.22	0.44	0.61
Tennessee	3.31	5.33	0.71	1.02	0.35	0.51
Texas	2.31	3.71	0.62	0.88	0.31	0.44
Utah	1.40	2.14	0.42	0.59	0.21	0.29
Vermont	2.72	4.15	0.85	1.17	0.42	0.58
Virginia	2.57	4.10	0.68	0.97	0.34	0.49
Washington	2.32	3.73	0.56	0.80	0.28	0.40
West Virginia	3.99	6.31	0.90	1.28	0.45	0.64
Wisconsin	2.74	4.40	0.61	0.87	0.30	0.44
Wyoming	3.30	5.03	0.94	1.28	0.47	0.64

Section C
Recommended Funding Levels, by State

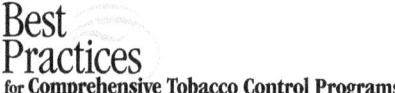

Section C: Recommended Funding Levels, by State

Alabama

Program Intervention Budgets — 2014

Recommended Annual Investment	$55.9 million
Deaths in State Caused by Smoking	
Annual average smoking-attributable deaths	7,600
Youth aged 0-17 projected to die from smoking	107,600
Annual Costs Incurred in State from Smoking	
Total medical	$1,886 million
State Revenue from Tobacco Sales and Settlement	
FY 2012 tobacco tax revenue	$134.6 million
FY 2012 tobacco settlement payment	$93.8 million
Total state revenue from tobacco sales and settlement	$228.4 million
Percent Tobacco Revenue to Fund at Recommended Level	**24%**

	Annual Total (Millions)		Annual Per Capita	
	Minimum	Recommended	Minimum	Recommended
I. State and Community Interventions Multiple social resources working together will have the greatest long-term population impact.	$14.4	$18.0	$2.99	$3.73
II. Mass-Reach Health Communication Interventions Media interventions work to prevent smoking initiation, promote cessation, and shape social norms.	$4.2	$6.0	$0.87	$1.24
III. Cessation Interventions Tobacco use treatment is effective and highly cost-effective.	$15.4	$24.6	$3.19	$5.10
IV. Surveillance and Evaluation Publicly funded programs should be accountable and demonstrate effectiveness.	$3.4	$4.9	$0.71	$1.01
V. Infrastructure, Administration, and Management Complex, integrated programs require experienced staff to provide fiscal management, accountability, and coordination.	$1.7	$2.4	$0.35	$0.50
TOTAL	$39.1	$55.9	$8.11	$11.58

Note: A justification for each program element and the rationale for the budget estimates are provided in Section A. The funding estimates presented are based on adjustments for changes in population and cost-of-living increases since *Best Practices — 2007* was published. The actual funding required for implementing programs will vary depending on state characteristics, such as prevalence of tobacco use, sociodemographic factors, and other factors. See Appendix E for data sources on deaths, costs, revenue, and state-specific factors.

Centers for Disease Control and Prevention • Office on Smoking and Health
www.cdc.gov/tobacco • tobaccoinfo@cdc.gov • 1 (800) CDC-INFO or 1 (800) 232-4636

Section C: Recommended Funding Levels, by State — **Best Practices for Comprehensive Tobacco Control Programs**

Alaska

Program Intervention Budgets — 2014

Recommended Annual Investment	$10.2 million
Deaths in State Caused by Smoking	
Annual average smoking-attributable deaths	500
Youth aged 0-17 projected to die from smoking	14,000
Annual Costs Incurred in State from Smoking	
Total medical	$ 438 million
State Revenue from Tobacco Sales and Settlement	
FY 2012 tobacco tax revenue	$ 71.3 million
FY 2012 tobacco settlement payment	$30.0 million
Total state revenue from tobacco sales and settlement	$101.3 million
Percent Tobacco Revenue to Fund at Recommended Level	10%

	Annual Total (Millions)		Annual Per Capita	
	Minimum	Recommended	Minimum	Recommended
I. State and Community Interventions Multiple social resources working together will have the greatest long-term population impact.	$3.3	$4.1	$4.51	$5.61
II. Mass-Reach Health Communication Interventions Media interventions work to prevent smoking initiation, promote cessation, and shape social norms.	$1.0	$1.4	$1.37	$1.91
III. Cessation Interventions Tobacco use treatment is effective and highly cost-effective.	$2.2	$3.4	$3.01	$4.65
IV. Surveillance and Evaluation Publicly funded programs should be accountable and demonstrate effectiveness.	$0.7	$0.9	$0.89	$1.22
V. Infrastructure, Administration, and Management Complex, integrated programs require experienced staff to provide fiscal management, accountability, and coordination.	$0.3	$0.4	$0.44	$0.61
TOTAL	$7.5	$10.2	$10.22	$14.00

Note: A justification for each program element and the rationale for the budget estimates are provided in Section A. The funding estimates presented are based on adjustments for changes in population and cost-of-living increases since *Best Practices — 2007* was published. The actual funding required for implementing programs will vary depending on state characteristics, such as prevalence of tobacco use, sociodemographic factors, and other factors. See Appendix E for data sources on deaths, costs, revenue, and state-specific factors.

Centers for Disease Control and Prevention • Office on Smoking and Health
www.cdc.gov/tobacco • tobaccoinfo@cdc.gov • 1 (800) CDC-INFO or 1 (800) 232-4636

Best Practices for Comprehensive Tobacco Control Programs

Section C: Recommended Funding Levels, by State

Arizona

Program Intervention Budgets — 2014

Recommended Annual Investment	$64.4 million
Deaths in State Caused by Smoking	
Annual average smoking-attributable deaths	7,100
Youth aged 0-17 projected to die from smoking	115,100
Annual Costs Incurred in State from Smoking	
Total medical	$2,383 million
State Revenue from Tobacco Sales and Settlement	
FY 2012 tobacco tax revenue	$337.8 million
FY 2012 tobacco settlement payment	$101.1 million
Total state revenue from tobacco sales and settlement	$438.9 million
Percent Tobacco Revenue to Fund at Recommended Level	**15%**

	Annual Total (Millions)		Annual Per Capita	
	Minimum	Recommended	Minimum	Recommended
I. State and Community Interventions Multiple social resources working together will have the greatest long-term population impact.	$16.8	$20.9	$2.56	$3.19
II. Mass-Reach Health Communication Interventions Media interventions work to prevent smoking initiation, promote cessation, and shape social norms.	$7.9	$11.4	$1.21	$1.74
III. Cessation Interventions Tobacco use treatment is effective and highly cost-effective.	$14.8	$23.7	$2.26	$3.62
IV. Surveillance and Evaluation Publicly funded programs should be accountable and demonstrate effectiveness.	$4.0	$5.6	$0.60	$0.86
V. Infrastructure, Administration, and Management Complex, integrated programs require experienced staff to provide fiscal management, accountability, and coordination.	$2.0	$2.8	$0.30	$0.43
TOTAL	$45.5	$64.4	$6.93	$9.84

Note: A justification for each program element and the rationale for the budget estimates are provided in Section A. The funding estimates presented are based on adjustments for changes in population and cost-of-living increases since *Best Practices — 2007* was published. The actual funding required for implementing programs will vary depending on state characteristics, such as prevalence of tobacco use, sociodemographic factors, and other factors. See Appendix E for data sources on deaths, costs, revenue, and state-specific factors.

Centers for Disease Control and Prevention • Office on Smoking and Health
www.cdc.gov/tobacco • tobaccoinfo@cdc.gov • 1 (800) CDC-INFO or 1 (800) 232-4636

Section C: Recommended Funding Levels, by State — **Best Practices for Comprehensive Tobacco Control Programs**

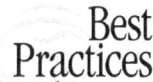

Arkansas

Program Intervention Budgets — 2014

Recommended Annual Investment	$36.7 million
Deaths in State Caused by Smoking	
Annual average smoking-attributable deaths	5,100
Youth aged 0-17 projected to die from smoking	68,700
Annual Costs Incurred in State from Smoking	
Total medical	$1,215 million
State Revenue from Tobacco Sales and Settlement	
FY 2012 tobacco tax revenue	$245.4 million
FY 2012 tobacco settlement payment	$50.5 million
Total state revenue from tobacco sales and settlement	$295.9 million
Percent Tobacco Revenue to Fund at Recommended Level	12%

	Annual Total (Millions)		Annual Per Capita	
	Minimum	Recommended	Minimum	Recommended
I. State and Community Interventions Multiple social resources working together will have the greatest long-term population impact.	$10.1	$12.7	$3.42	$4.31
II. Mass-Reach Health Communication Interventions Media interventions work to prevent smoking initiation, promote cessation, and shape social norms.	$2.5	$3.5	$0.85	$1.19
III. Cessation Interventions Tobacco use treatment is effective and highly cost-effective.	$9.9	$15.7	$3.36	$5.32
IV. Surveillance and Evaluation Publicly funded programs should be accountable and demonstrate effectiveness.	$2.3	$3.2	$0.76	$1.08
V. Infrastructure, Administration, and Management Complex, integrated programs require experienced staff to provide fiscal management, accountability, and coordination.	$1.1	$1.6	$0.38	$0.54
TOTAL	$25.9	$36.7	$8.77	$12.44

Note: A justification for each program element and the rationale for the budget estimates are provided in Section A. The funding estimates presented are based on adjustments for changes in population and cost-of-living increases since *Best Practices — 2007* was published. The actual funding required for implementing programs will vary depending on state characteristics, such as prevalence of tobacco use, sociodemographic factors, and other factors. See Appendix E for data sources on deaths, costs, revenue, and state-specific factors.

Centers for Disease Control and Prevention • Office on Smoking and Health
www.cdc.gov/tobacco • tobaccoinfo@cdc.gov • 1 (800) CDC-INFO or 1 (800) 232-4636

Best Practices for Comprehensive Tobacco Control Programs

Section C: Recommended Funding Levels, by State

California

Program Intervention Budgets — 2014

Recommended Annual Investment	$347.9 million
Deaths in State Caused by Smoking	
Annual average smoking-attributable deaths	33,900
Youth aged 0-17 projected to die from smoking	440,600
Annual Costs Incurred in State from Smoking	
Total medical	$13,292 million
State Revenue from Tobacco Sales and Settlement	
FY 2012 tobacco tax revenue	$891.1 million
FY 2012 tobacco settlement payment	$735.8 million
Total state revenue from tobacco sales and settlement	$1,626.9 million
Percent Tobacco Revenue to Fund at Recommended Level	**21%**

	Annual Total (Millions)		Annual Per Capita	
	Minimum	Recommended	Minimum	Recommended
I. State and Community Interventions Multiple social resources working together will have the greatest long-term population impact.	$99.9	$124.9	$2.63	$3.28
II. Mass-Reach Health Communication Interventions Media interventions work to prevent smoking initiation, promote cessation, and shape social norms.	$52.8	$76.0	$1.39	$2.00
III. Cessation Interventions Tobacco use treatment is effective and highly cost-effective.	$63.5	$101.6	$1.67	$2.67
IV. Surveillance and Evaluation Publicly funded programs should be accountable and demonstrate effectiveness.	$21.6	$30.3	$0.57	$0.80
V. Infrastructure, Administration, and Management Complex, integrated programs require experienced staff to provide fiscal management, accountability, and coordination.	$10.8	$15.1	$0.28	$0.40
TOTAL	$248.6	$347.9	$6.54	$9.15

Note: A justification for each program element and the rationale for the budget estimates are provided in Section A. The funding estimates presented are based on adjustments for changes in population and cost-of-living increases since *Best Practices — 2007* was published. The actual funding required for implementing programs will vary depending on state characteristics, such as prevalence of tobacco use, sociodemographic factors, and other factors. See Appendix E for data sources on deaths, costs, revenue, and state-specific factors.

Centers for Disease Control and Prevention • Office on Smoking and Health
www.cdc.gov/tobacco • tobaccoinfo@cdc.gov • 1 (800) CDC-INFO or 1 (800) 232-4636

Section C: Recommended Funding Levels, by State — Best Practices for Comprehensive Tobacco Control Programs

Colorado

Program Intervention Budgets — 2014

Recommended Annual Investment	$52.9 million
Deaths in State Caused by Smoking	
Annual average smoking-attributable deaths	4,400
Youth aged 0-17 projected to die from smoking	90,600
Annual Costs Incurred in State from Smoking	
Total medical	$1,891 million
State Revenue from Tobacco Sales and Settlement	
FY 2012 tobacco tax revenue	$203.4 million
FY 2012 tobacco settlement payment	$90.8 million
Total state revenue from tobacco sales and settlement	$294.2 million
Percent Tobacco Revenue to Fund at Recommended Level	18%

	Annual Total (Millions)		Annual Per Capita	
	Minimum	Recommended	Minimum	Recommended
I. State and Community Interventions Multiple social resources working together will have the greatest long-term population impact.	$13.2	$16.4	$2.54	$3.16
II. Mass-Reach Health Communication Interventions Media interventions work to prevent smoking initiation, promote cessation, and shape social norms.	$6.9	$9.9	$1.33	$1.91
III. Cessation Interventions Tobacco use treatment is effective and highly cost-effective.	$12.4	$19.7	$2.39	$3.80
IV. Surveillance and Evaluation Publicly funded programs should be accountable and demonstrate effectiveness.	$3.3	$4.6	$0.63	$0.89
V. Infrastructure, Administration, and Management Complex, integrated programs require experienced staff to provide fiscal management, accountability, and coordination.	$1.6	$2.3	$0.31	$0.44
TOTAL	$37.4	$52.9	$7.20	$10.20

Note: A justification for each program element and the rationale for the budget estimates are provided in Section A. The funding estimates presented are based on adjustments for changes in population and cost-of-living increases since *Best Practices—2007* was published. The actual funding required for implementing programs will vary depending on state characteristics, such as prevalence of tobacco use, sociodemographic factors, and other factors. See Appendix E for data sources on deaths, costs, revenue, and state-specific factors.

Centers for Disease Control and Prevention • Office on Smoking and Health
www.cdc.gov/tobacco • tobaccoinfo@cdc.gov • 1 (800) CDC-INFO or 1 (800) 232-4636

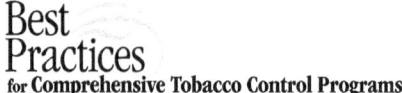

Connecticut

Program Intervention Budgets — 2014

Recommended Annual Investment	$32.0 million
Deaths in State Caused by Smoking	
Annual average smoking-attributable deaths	4,300
Youth aged 0-17 projected to die from smoking	56,100
Annual Costs Incurred in State from Smoking	
Total medical	$2,039 million
State Revenue from Tobacco Sales and Settlement	
FY 2012 tobacco tax revenue	$418.2 million
FY 2012 tobacco settlement payment	$123.8 million
Total state revenue from tobacco sales and settlement	$542.0 million
Percent Tobacco Revenue to Fund at Recommended Level	6%

	Annual Total (Millions)		Annual Per Capita	
	Minimum	Recommended	Minimum	Recommended
I. State and Community Interventions Multiple social resources working together will have the greatest long-term population impact.	$9.1	$11.4	$2.53	$3.18
II. Mass-Reach Health Communication Interventions Media interventions work to prevent smoking initiation, promote cessation, and shape social norms.	$2.6	$3.7	$0.72	$1.03
III. Cessation Interventions Tobacco use treatment is effective and highly cost-effective.	$8.0	$12.7	$2.23	$3.54
IV. Surveillance and Evaluation Publicly funded programs should be accountable and demonstrate effectiveness.	$2.0	$2.8	$0.55	$0.78
V. Infrastructure, Administration, and Management Complex, integrated programs require experienced staff to provide fiscal management, accountability, and coordination.	$1.0	$1.4	$0.27	$0.39
TOTAL	$22.7	$32.0	$6.30	$8.92

Note: A justification for each program element and the rationale for the budget estimates are provided in Section A. The funding estimates presented are based on adjustments for changes in population and cost-of-living increases since *Best Practices — 2007* was published. The actual funding required for implementing programs will vary depending on state characteristics, such as prevalence of tobacco use, sociodemographic factors, and other factors. See Appendix E for data sources on deaths, costs, revenue, and state-specific factors.

Centers for Disease Control and Prevention • Office on Smoking and Health
www.cdc.gov/tobacco • tobaccoinfo@cdc.gov • 1 (800) CDC-INFO or 1 (800) 232-4636

Section C: Recommended Funding Levels, by State — **Best Practices for Comprehensive Tobacco Control Programs**

Delaware

Program Intervention Budgets — 2014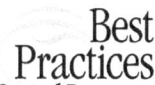

Recommended Annual Investment	$13.0 million
Deaths in State Caused by Smoking	
Annual average smoking-attributable deaths	1,300
Youth aged 0-17 projected to die from smoking	17,200
Annual Costs Incurred in State from Smoking	
Total medical	$532 million
State Revenue from Tobacco Sales and Settlement	
FY 2012 tobacco tax revenue	$126.0 million
FY 2012 tobacco settlement payment	$26.7 million
Total state revenue from tobacco sales and settlement	$152.7 million
Percent Tobacco Revenue to Fund at Recommended Level	9%

	Annual Total (Millions)		Annual Per Capita	
	Minimum	Recommended	Minimum	Recommended
I. State and Community Interventions Multiple social resources working together will have the greatest long-term population impact.	$3.4	$4.3	$3.71	$4.69
II. Mass-Reach Health Communication Interventions Media interventions work to prevent smoking initiation, promote cessation, and shape social norms.	$2.0	$2.8	$2.18	$3.05
III. Cessation Interventions Tobacco use treatment is effective and highly cost-effective.	$2.7	$4.2	$2.94	$4.58
IV. Surveillance and Evaluation Publicly funded programs should be accountable and demonstrate effectiveness.	$0.8	$1.1	$0.88	$1.23
V. Infrastructure, Administration, and Management Complex, integrated programs require experienced staff to provide fiscal management, accountability, and coordination.	$0.4	$0.6	$0.44	$0.62
TOTAL	$9.3	$13.0	$10.15	$14.17

Note: A justification for each program element and the rationale for the budget estimates are provided in Section A. The funding estimates presented are based on adjustments for changes in population and cost-of-living increases since *Best Practices—2007* was published. The actual funding required for implementing programs will vary depending on state characteristics, such as prevalence of tobacco use, sociodemographic factors, and other factors. See Appendix E for data sources on deaths, costs, revenue, and state-specific factors.

Centers for Disease Control and Prevention • Office on Smoking and Health
www.cdc.gov/tobacco • tobaccoinfo@cdc.gov • 1 (800) CDC-INFO or 1 (800) 232-4636

District of Columbia

Program Intervention Budgets — 2014

Recommended Annual Investment	**$10.7 million**
Deaths in State Caused by Smoking	
Annual average smoking-attributable deaths	700
Youth aged 0-17 projected to die from smoking	7,100
Annual Costs Incurred in State from Smoking	
Total medical	$391 million
State Revenue from Tobacco Sales and Settlement	
FY 2012 tobacco tax revenue	$34.1 million
FY 2012 tobacco settlement payment	$38.3 million
Total state revenue from tobacco sales and settlement	$72.4 million
Percent Tobacco Revenue to Fund at Recommended Level	**15%**

	Annual Total (Millions)		Annual Per Capita	
	Minimum	Recommended	Minimum	Recommended
I. State and Community Interventions Multiple social resources working together will have the greatest long-term population impact.	$3.4	$4.2	$5.38	$6.64
II. Mass-Reach Health Communication Interventions Media interventions work to prevent smoking initiation, promote cessation, and shape social norms.	$1.4	$2.0	$2.21	$3.16
III. Cessation Interventions Tobacco use treatment is effective and highly cost-effective.	$2.0	$3.1	$3.16	$4.90
IV. Surveillance and Evaluation Publicly funded programs should be accountable and demonstrate effectiveness.	$0.7	$0.9	$1.08	$1.47
V. Infrastructure, Administration, and Management Complex, integrated programs require experienced staff to provide fiscal management, accountability, and coordination.	$0.3	$0.5	$0.54	$0.74
TOTAL	$7.8	$10.7	$12.37	$16.91

Note: A justification for each program element and the rationale for the budget estimates are provided in Section A. The funding estimates presented are based on adjustments for changes in population and cost-of-living increases since *Best Practices — 2007* was published. The actual funding required for implementing programs will vary depending on state characteristics, such as prevalence of tobacco use, sociodemographic factors, and other factors. See Appendix E for data sources on deaths, costs, revenue, and state-specific factors.

Centers for Disease Control and Prevention • Office on Smoking and Health
www.cdc.gov/tobacco • tobaccoinfo@cdc.gov • 1 (800) CDC-INFO or 1 (800) 232-4636

Section C: Recommended Funding Levels, by State — **Best Practices** for Comprehensive Tobacco Control Programs

Florida

Program Intervention Budgets — 2014

Recommended Annual Investment	**$194.2 million**
Deaths in State Caused by Smoking	
Annual average smoking-attributable deaths	28,100
Youth aged 0-17 projected to die from smoking	270,200
Annual Costs Incurred in State from Smoking	
Total medical	$8,644 million
State Revenue from Tobacco Sales and Settlement	
FY 2012 tobacco tax revenue	$1,238.0 million
FY 2012 tobacco settlement payment	$383.0 million
Total state revenue from tobacco sales and settlement	$1,621.0 million
Percent Tobacco Revenue to Fund at Recommended Level	**12%**

	Annual Total (Millions)		Annual Per Capita	
	Minimum	Recommended	Minimum	Recommended
I. State and Community Interventions Multiple social resources working together will have the greatest long-term population impact.	$44.9	$56.2	$2.32	$2.91
II. Mass-Reach Health Communication Interventions Media interventions work to prevent smoking initiation, promote cessation, and shape social norms.	$25.9	$37.2	$1.34	$1.93
III. Cessation Interventions Tobacco use treatment is effective and highly cost-effective.	$47.0	$75.5	$2.43	$3.91
IV. Surveillance and Evaluation Publicly funded programs should be accountable and demonstrate effectiveness.	$11.8	$16.9	$0.61	$0.88
V. Infrastructure, Administration, and Management Complex, integrated programs require experienced staff to provide fiscal management, accountability, and coordination.	$5.9	$8.4	$0.30	$0.44
TOTAL	$135.5	$194.2	$7.00	$10.07

Note: A justification for each program element and the rationale for the budget estimates are provided in Section A. The funding estimates presented are based on adjustments for changes in population and cost-of-living increases since *Best Practices—2007* was published. The actual funding required for implementing programs will vary depending on state characteristics, such as prevalence of tobacco use, sociodemographic factors, and other factors. See Appendix E for data sources on deaths, costs, revenue, and state-specific factors.

Centers for Disease Control and Prevention • Office on Smoking and Health
www.cdc.gov/tobacco • tobaccoinfo@cdc.gov • 1 (800) CDC-INFO or 1 (800) 232-4636

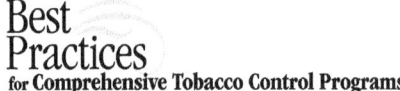

Section C: Recommended Funding Levels, by State

Georgia

Program Intervention Budgets — 2014

Recommended Annual Investment	**$106.0 million**
Deaths in State Caused by Smoking	
Annual average smoking-attributable deaths	10,300
Youth aged 0-17 projected to die from smoking	204,000
Annual Costs Incurred in State from Smoking	
Total medical	$3,183 million
State Revenue from Tobacco Sales and Settlement	
FY 2012 tobacco tax revenue	$225.0 million
FY 2012 tobacco settlement payment	$141.1 million
Total state revenue from tobacco sales and settlement	$366.1 million
Percent Tobacco Revenue to Fund at Recommended Level	**29%**

	Annual Total (Millions)		Annual Per Capita	
	Minimum	Recommended	Minimum	Recommended
I. State and Community Interventions Multiple social resources working together will have the greatest long-term population impact.	$28.0	$35.0	$2.82	$3.53
II. Mass-Reach Health Communication Interventions Media interventions work to prevent smoking initiation, promote cessation, and shape social norms.	$10.4	$14.9	$1.05	$1.50
III. Cessation Interventions Tobacco use treatment is effective and highly cost-effective.	$26.3	$42.3	$2.65	$4.26
IV. Surveillance and Evaluation Publicly funded programs should be accountable and demonstrate effectiveness.	$6.5	$9.2	$0.65	$0.93
V. Infrastructure, Administration, and Management Complex, integrated programs require experienced staff to provide fiscal management, accountability, and coordination.	$3.2	$4.6	$0.33	$0.46
TOTAL	$74.4	$106.0	$7.50	$10.68

Note: A justification for each program element and the rationale for the budget estimates are provided in Section A. The funding estimates presented are based on adjustments for changes in population and cost-of-living increases since *Best Practices—2007* was published. The actual funding required for implementing programs will vary depending on state characteristics, such as prevalence of tobacco use, sociodemographic factors, and other factors. See Appendix E for data sources on deaths, costs, revenue, and state-specific factors.

Centers for Disease Control and Prevention • Office on Smoking and Health
www.cdc.gov/tobacco • tobaccoinfo@cdc.gov • 1 (800) CDC-INFO or 1 (800) 232-4636

Section C: Recommended Funding Levels, by State — **Best Practices** for Comprehensive Tobacco Control Programs

Hawaii

Program Intervention Budgets — 2014

Recommended Annual Investment	**$13.7 million**
Deaths in State Caused by Smoking	
Annual average smoking-attributable deaths	1,200
Youth aged 0-17 projected to die from smoking	21,400
Annual Costs Incurred in State from Smoking	
Total medical	$526 million
State Revenue from Tobacco Sales and Settlement	
FY 2012 tobacco tax revenue	$138.8 million
FY 2012 tobacco settlement payment	$48.6 million
Total state revenue from tobacco sales and settlement	$187.4 million
Percent Tobacco Revenue to Fund at Recommended Level	**7%**

	Annual Total (Millions)		Annual Per Capita	
	Minimum	Recommended	Minimum	Recommended
I. State and Community Interventions Multiple social resources working together will have the greatest long-term population impact.	$4.5	$5.6	$3.23	$4.02
II. Mass-Reach Health Communication Interventions Media interventions work to prevent smoking initiation, promote cessation, and shape social norms.	$1.1	$1.6	$0.79	$1.15
III. Cessation Interventions Tobacco use treatment is effective and highly cost-effective.	$3.0	$4.7	$2.15	$3.38
IV. Surveillance and Evaluation Publicly funded programs should be accountable and demonstrate effectiveness.	$0.9	$1.2	$0.62	$0.86
V. Infrastructure, Administration, and Management Complex, integrated programs require experienced staff to provide fiscal management, accountability, and coordination.	$0.4	$0.6	$0.31	$0.43
TOTAL	$9.9	$13.7	$7.10	$9.84

Note: A justification for each program element and the rationale for the budget estimates are provided in Section A. The funding estimates presented are based on adjustments for changes in population and cost-of-living increases since *Best Practices—2007* was published. The actual funding required for implementing programs will vary depending on state characteristics, such as prevalence of tobacco use, sociodemographic factors, and other factors. See Appendix E for data sources on deaths, costs, revenue, and state-specific factors.

Centers for Disease Control and Prevention • Office on Smoking and Health
www.cdc.gov/tobacco • tobaccoinfo@cdc.gov • 1 (800) CDC-INFO or 1 (800) 232-4636

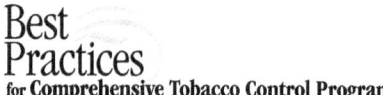

Idaho

Program Intervention Budgets — 2014

Recommended Annual Investment	$15.6 million
Deaths in State Caused by Smoking	
Annual average smoking-attributable deaths	1,600
Youth aged 0-17 projected to die from smoking	30,200
Annual Costs Incurred in State from Smoking	
Total medical	$508 million
State Revenue from Tobacco Sales and Settlement	
FY 2012 tobacco tax revenue	$48.3 million
FY 2012 tobacco settlement payment	$24.9 million
Total state revenue from tobacco sales and settlement	$73.2 million
Percent Tobacco Revenue to Fund at Recommended Level	21%

	Annual Total (Millions)		Annual Per Capita	
	Minimum	Recommended	Minimum	Recommended
I. State and Community Interventions Multiple social resources working together will have the greatest long-term population impact.	$4.7	$5.8	$2.95	$3.63
II. Mass-Reach Health Communication Interventions Media interventions work to prevent smoking initiation, promote cessation, and shape social norms.	$1.5	$2.1	$0.94	$1.32
III. Cessation Interventions Tobacco use treatment is effective and highly cost-effective.	$3.6	$5.6	$2.26	$3.51
IV. Surveillance and Evaluation Publicly funded programs should be accountable and demonstrate effectiveness.	$1.0	$1.4	$0.62	$0.85
V. Infrastructure, Administration, and Management Complex, integrated programs require experienced staff to provide fiscal management, accountability, and coordination.	$0.5	$0.7	$0.31	$0.42
TOTAL	$11.3	$15.6	$7.08	$9.73

Note: A justification for each program element and the rationale for the budget estimates are provided in Section A. The funding estimates presented are based on adjustments for changes in population and cost-of-living increases since *Best Practices — 2007* was published. The actual funding required for implementing programs will vary depending on state characteristics, such as prevalence of tobacco use, sociodemographic factors, and other factors. See Appendix E for data sources on deaths, costs, revenue, and state-specific factors.

Centers for Disease Control and Prevention • Office on Smoking and Health
www.cdc.gov/tobacco • tobaccoinfo@cdc.gov • 1 (800) CDC-INFO or 1 (800) 232-4636

Section C: Recommended Funding Levels, by State — **Best Practices** for **Comprehensive Tobacco Control Programs**

Illinois

Program Intervention Budgets — 2014

Recommended Annual Investment	$136.7 million
Deaths in State Caused by Smoking	
Annual average smoking-attributable deaths	16,000
Youth aged 0-17 projected to die from smoking	230,400
Annual Costs Incurred in State from Smoking	
Total medical	$5,496 million
State Revenue from Tobacco Sales and Settlement	
FY 2012 tobacco tax revenue	$608.8 million
FY 2012 tobacco settlement payment	$273.7 million
Total state revenue from tobacco sales and settlement	$882.5 million
Percent Tobacco Revenue to Fund at Recommended Level	15%

	Annual Total (Millions)		Annual Per Capita	
	Minimum	Recommended	Minimum	Recommended
I. State and Community Interventions Multiple social resources working together will have the greatest long-term population impact.	$36.1	$45.2	$2.80	$3.51
II. Mass-Reach Health Communication Interventions Media interventions work to prevent smoking initiation, promote cessation, and shape social norms.	$15.9	$22.8	$1.23	$1.77
III. Cessation Interventions Tobacco use treatment is effective and highly cost-effective.	$31.7	$50.9	$2.46	$3.95
IV. Surveillance and Evaluation Publicly funded programs should be accountable and demonstrate effectiveness.	$8.4	$11.9	$0.65	$0.92
V. Infrastructure, Administration, and Management Complex, integrated programs require experienced staff to provide fiscal management, accountability, and coordination.	$4.2	$5.9	$0.32	$0.46
TOTAL	$96.3	$136.7	$7.46	$10.61

Note: A justification for each program element and the rationale for the budget estimates are provided in Section A. The funding estimates presented are based on adjustments for changes in population and cost-of-living increases since Best Practices — 2007 was published. The actual funding required for implementing programs will vary depending on state characteristics, such as prevalence of tobacco use, sociodemographic factors, and other factors. See Appendix E for data sources on deaths, costs, revenue, and state-specific factors.

Centers for Disease Control and Prevention • Office on Smoking and Health
www.cdc.gov/tobacco • tobaccoinfo@cdc.gov • 1 (800) CDC-INFO or 1 (800) 232-4636

Best Practices for Comprehensive Tobacco Control Programs

Section C: Recommended Funding Levels, by State

Indiana

Program Intervention Budgets — 2014

Recommended Annual Investment	$73.5 million
Deaths in State Caused by Smoking	
Annual average smoking-attributable deaths	9,800
Youth aged 0-17 projected to die from smoking	150,700
Annual Costs Incurred in State from Smoking	
Total medical	$2,930 million
State Revenue from Tobacco Sales and Settlement	
FY 2012 tobacco tax revenue	$457.2 million
FY 2012 tobacco settlement payment	$129.5 million
Total state revenue from tobacco sales and settlement	$586.7 million
Percent Tobacco Revenue to Fund at Recommended Level	**13%**

	Annual Total (Millions)		Annual Per Capita	
	Minimum	Recommended	Minimum	Recommended
I. State and Community Interventions Multiple social resources working together will have the greatest long-term population impact.	$18.8	$23.5	$2.88	$3.59
II. Mass-Reach Health Communication Interventions Media interventions work to prevent smoking initiation, promote cessation, and shape social norms.	$5.1	$7.3	$0.78	$1.12
III. Cessation Interventions Tobacco use treatment is effective and highly cost-effective.	$20.6	$33.1	$3.15	$5.06
IV. Surveillance and Evaluation Publicly funded programs should be accountable and demonstrate effectiveness.	$4.5	$6.4	$0.68	$0.98
V. Infrastructure, Administration, and Management Complex, integrated programs require experienced staff to provide fiscal management, accountability, and coordination.	$2.2	$3.2	$0.34	$0.49
TOTAL	$51.2	$73.5	$7.83	$11.24

Note: A justification for each program element and the rationale for the budget estimates are provided in Section A. The funding estimates presented are based on adjustments for changes in population and cost-of-living increases since *Best Practices—2007* was published. The actual funding required for implementing programs will vary depending on state characteristics, such as prevalence of tobacco use, sociodemographic factors, and other factors. See Appendix E for data sources on deaths, costs, revenue, and state-specific factors.

Centers for Disease Control and Prevention • Office on Smoking and Health
www.cdc.gov/tobacco • tobaccoinfo@cdc.gov • 1 (800) CDC-INFO or 1 (800) 232-4636

Section C: Recommended Funding Levels, by State — **Best Practices** for Comprehensive Tobacco Control Programs

Iowa

Program Intervention Budgets — 2014

Recommended Annual Investment	**$30.1 million**
Deaths in State Caused by Smoking	
Annual average smoking-attributable deaths	4,500
Youth aged 0-17 projected to die from smoking	55,100
Annual Costs Incurred in State from Smoking	
Total medical	$1,285 million
State Revenue from Tobacco Sales and Settlement	
FY 2012 tobacco tax revenue	$225.4 million
FY 2012 tobacco settlement payment	$65.7 million
Total state revenue from tobacco sales and settlement	$291.1 million
Percent Tobacco Revenue to Fund at Recommended Level	**10%**

	Annual Total (Millions)		Annual Per Capita	
	Minimum	Recommended	Minimum	Recommended
I. State and Community Interventions Multiple social resources working together will have the greatest long-term population impact.	$8.4	$10.5	$2.73	$3.42
II. Mass-Reach Health Communication Interventions Media interventions work to prevent smoking initiation, promote cessation, and shape social norms.	$2.5	$3.6	$0.81	$1.17
III. Cessation Interventions Tobacco use treatment is effective and highly cost-effective.	$7.6	$12.1	$2.47	$3.94
IV. Surveillance and Evaluation Publicly funded programs should be accountable and demonstrate effectiveness.	$1.9	$2.6	$0.60	$0.85
V. Infrastructure, Administration, and Management Complex, integrated programs require experienced staff to provide fiscal management, accountability, and coordination.	$0.9	$1.3	$0.30	$0.43
TOTAL	$21.3	$30.1	$6.91	$9.81

Note: A justification for each program element and the rationale for the budget estimates are provided in Section A. The funding estimates presented are based on adjustments for changes in population and cost-of-living increases since *Best Practices—2007* was published. The actual funding required for implementing programs will vary depending on state characteristics, such as prevalence of tobacco use, sociodemographic factors, and other factors. See Appendix E for data sources on deaths, costs, revenue, and state-specific factors.

Centers for Disease Control and Prevention • Office on Smoking and Health
www.cdc.gov/tobacco • tobaccoinfo@cdc.gov • 1 (800) CDC-INFO or 1 (800) 232-4636

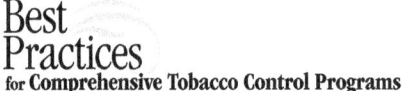

Section C: Recommended Funding Levels, by State

Kansas

Program Intervention Budgets — 2014

Recommended Annual Investment	$27.9 million
Deaths in State Caused by Smoking	
Annual average smoking-attributable deaths	3,800
Youth aged 0-17 projected to die from smoking	61,200
Annual Costs Incurred in State from Smoking	
Total medical	$1,128 million
State Revenue from Tobacco Sales and Settlement	
FY 2012 tobacco tax revenue	$103.9 million
FY 2012 tobacco settlement payment	$58.0 million
Total state revenue from tobacco sales and settlement	$161.9 million
Percent Tobacco Revenue to Fund at Recommended Level	**17%**

	Annual Total (Millions)		Annual Per Capita	
	Minimum	Recommended	Minimum	Recommended
I. State and Community Interventions Multiple social resources working together will have the greatest long-term population impact.	$8.4	$10.5	$2.91	$3.64
II. Mass-Reach Health Communication Interventions Media interventions work to prevent smoking initiation, promote cessation, and shape social norms.	$1.3	$1.9	$0.45	$0.66
III. Cessation Interventions Tobacco use treatment is effective and highly cost-effective.	$7.5	$11.9	$2.60	$4.12
IV. Surveillance and Evaluation Publicly funded programs should be accountable and demonstrate effectiveness.	$1.7	$2.4	$0.60	$0.84
V. Infrastructure, Administration, and Management Complex, integrated programs require experienced staff to provide fiscal management, accountability, and coordination.	$0.9	$1.2	$0.30	$0.42
TOTAL	$19.8	$27.9	$6.86	$9.68

Note: A justification for each program element and the rationale for the budget estimates are provided in Section A. The funding estimates presented are based on adjustments for changes in population and cost-of-living increases since *Best Practices — 2007* was published. The actual funding required for implementing programs will vary depending on state characteristics, such as prevalence of tobacco use, sociodemographic factors, and other factors. See Appendix E for data sources on deaths, costs, revenue, and state-specific factors.

Centers for Disease Control and Prevention • Office on Smoking and Health
www.cdc.gov/tobacco • tobaccoinfo@cdc.gov • 1 (800) CDC-INFO or 1 (800) 232-4636

Section C: Recommended Funding Levels, by State — **Best Practices** for Comprehensive Tobacco Control Programs

Kentucky

Program Intervention Budgets — 2014

Recommended Annual Investment	$56.4 million
Deaths in State Caused by Smoking	
Annual average smoking-attributable deaths	7,900
Youth aged 0-17 projected to die from smoking	118,900
Annual Costs Incurred in State from Smoking	
Total medical	$1,927 million
State Revenue from Tobacco Sales and Settlement	
FY 2012 tobacco tax revenue	$282.9 million
FY 2012 tobacco settlement payment	$101.8 million
Total state revenue from tobacco sales and settlement	$384.7 million
Percent Tobacco Revenue to Fund at Recommended Level	15%

	Annual Total (Millions)		Annual Per Capita	
	Minimum	Recommended	Minimum	Recommended
I. State and Community Interventions Multiple social resources working together will have the greatest long-term population impact.	$15.2	$19.0	$3.47	$4.34
II. Mass-Reach Health Communication Interventions Media interventions work to prevent smoking initiation, promote cessation, and shape social norms.	$2.4	$3.5	$0.55	$0.80
III. Cessation Interventions Tobacco use treatment is effective and highly cost-effective.	$16.5	$26.5	$3.77	$6.05
IV. Surveillance and Evaluation Publicly funded programs should be accountable and demonstrate effectiveness.	$3.4	$4.9	$0.78	$1.12
V. Infrastructure, Administration, and Management Complex, integrated programs require experienced staff to provide fiscal management, accountability, and coordination.	$1.7	$2.5	$0.39	$0.56
TOTAL	$39.2	$56.4	$8.96	$12.87

Note: A justification for each program element and the rationale for the budget estimates are provided in Section A. The funding estimates presented are based on adjustments for changes in population and cost-of-living increases since Best Practices — 2007 was published. The actual funding required for implementing programs will vary depending on state characteristics, such as prevalence of tobacco use, sociodemographic factors, and other factors. See Appendix E for data sources on deaths, costs, revenue, and state-specific factors.

Centers for Disease Control and Prevention • Office on Smoking and Health
www.cdc.gov/tobacco • tobaccoinfo@cdc.gov • 1 (800) CDC-INFO or 1 (800) 232-4636

Best Practices for Comprehensive Tobacco Control Programs

Section C: Recommended Funding Levels, by State

Louisiana

Program Intervention Budgets — 2014

Recommended Annual Investment	$59.6 million
Deaths in State Caused by Smoking	
Annual average smoking-attributable deaths	6,200
Youth aged 0-17 projected to die from smoking	98,400
Annual Costs Incurred in State from Smoking	
Total medical	$1,892 million
State Revenue from Tobacco Sales and Settlement	
FY 2012 tobacco tax revenue	$140.0 million
FY 2012 tobacco settlement payment	$141.2 million
Total state revenue from tobacco sales and settlement	$281.2 million
Percent Tobacco Revenue to Fund at Recommended Level	**21%**

	Annual Total (Millions)		Annual Per Capita	
	Minimum	Recommended	Minimum	Recommended
I. State and Community Interventions Multiple social resources working together will have the greatest long-term population impact.	$15.6	$19.5	$3.39	$4.24
II. Mass-Reach Health Communication Interventions Media interventions work to prevent smoking initiation, promote cessation, and shape social norms.	$5.7	$8.1	$1.24	$1.76
III. Cessation Interventions Tobacco use treatment is effective and highly cost-effective.	$15.1	$24.2	$3.28	$5.26
IV. Surveillance and Evaluation Publicly funded programs should be accountable and demonstrate effectiveness.	$3.6	$5.2	$0.79	$1.13
V. Infrastructure, Administration, and Management Complex, integrated programs require experienced staff to provide fiscal management, accountability, and coordination.	$1.8	$2.6	$0.40	$0.56
TOTAL	$41.8	$59.6	$9.10	$12.95

Note: A justification for each program element and the rationale for the budget estimates are provided in Section A. The funding estimates presented are based on adjustments for changes in population and cost-of-living increases since *Best Practices — 2007* was published. The actual funding required for implementing programs will vary depending on state characteristics, such as prevalence of tobacco use, sociodemographic factors, and other factors. See Appendix E for data sources on deaths, costs, revenue, and state-specific factors.

Centers for Disease Control and Prevention • Office on Smoking and Health
www.cdc.gov/tobacco • tobaccoinfo@cdc.gov • 1 (800) CDC-INFO or 1 (800) 232-4636

Section C: Recommended Funding Levels, by State — 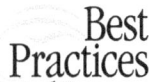 **Best Practices** for Comprehensive Tobacco Control Programs

Maine

Program Intervention Budgets — 2014

Recommended Annual Investment	$15.9 million
Deaths in State Caused by Smoking	
Annual average smoking-attributable deaths	2,200
Youth aged 0-17 projected to die from smoking	27,000
Annual Costs Incurred in State from Smoking	
Total medical	$811 million
State Revenue from Tobacco Sales and Settlement	
FY 2012 tobacco tax revenue	$139.7 million
FY 2012 tobacco settlement payment	$51.0 million
Total state revenue from tobacco sales and settlement	$190.7 million
Percent Tobacco Revenue to Fund at Recommended Level	8%

	Annual Total (Millions)		Annual Per Capita	
	Minimum	Recommended	Minimum	Recommended
I. State and Community Interventions Multiple social resources working together will have the greatest long-term population impact.	$4.1	$5.2	$3.08	$3.91
II. Mass-Reach Health Communication Interventions Media interventions work to prevent smoking initiation, promote cessation, and shape social norms.	$1.6	$2.3	$1.20	$1.73
III. Cessation Interventions Tobacco use treatment is effective and highly cost-effective.	$4.0	$6.3	$3.01	$4.74
IV. Surveillance and Evaluation Publicly funded programs should be accountable and demonstrate effectiveness.	$1.0	$1.4	$0.73	$1.04
V. Infrastructure, Administration, and Management Complex, integrated programs require experienced staff to provide fiscal management, accountability, and coordination.	$0.5	$0.7	$0.36	$0.52
TOTAL	$11.2	$15.9	$8.38	$11.94

Note: A justification for each program element and the rationale for the budget estimates are provided in Section A. The funding estimates presented are based on adjustments for changes in population and cost-of-living increases since *Best Practices—2007* was published. The actual funding required for implementing programs will vary depending on state characteristics, such as prevalence of tobacco use, sociodemographic factors, and other factors. See Appendix E for data sources on deaths, costs, revenue, and state-specific factors.

Centers for Disease Control and Prevention • Office on Smoking and Health
www.cdc.gov/tobacco • tobaccoinfo@cdc.gov • 1 (800) CDC-INFO or 1 (800) 232-4636

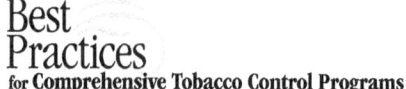

Section C: Recommended Funding Levels, by State

Maryland

Program Intervention Budgets — 2014

Recommended Annual Investment	$48.0 million
Deaths in State Caused by Smoking	
Annual average smoking-attributable deaths	6,400
Youth aged 0-17 projected to die from smoking	92,500
Annual Costs Incurred in State from Smoking	
Total medical	$2,710 million
State Revenue from Tobacco Sales and Settlement	
FY 2012 tobacco tax revenue	$410.7 million
FY 2012 tobacco settlement payment	$145.8 million
Total state revenue from tobacco sales and settlement	$556.5 million
Percent Tobacco Revenue to Fund at Recommended Level	9%

	Annual Total (Millions)		Annual Per Capita	
	Minimum	Recommended	Minimum	Recommended
I. State and Community Interventions Multiple social resources working together will have the greatest long-term population impact.	$12.8	$16.0	$2.18	$2.72
II. Mass-Reach Health Communication Interventions Media interventions work to prevent smoking initiation, promote cessation, and shape social norms.	$3.5	$5.0	$0.59	$0.85
III. Cessation Interventions Tobacco use treatment is effective and highly cost-effective.	$13.0	$20.7	$2.21	$3.52
IV. Surveillance and Evaluation Publicly funded programs should be accountable and demonstrate effectiveness.	$2.9	$4.2	$0.50	$0.71
V. Infrastructure, Administration, and Management Complex, integrated programs require experienced staff to provide fiscal management, accountability, and coordination.	$1.5	$2.1	$0.25	$0.35
TOTAL	$33.7	$48.0	$5.73	$8.15

Note: A justification for each program element and the rationale for the budget estimates are provided in Section A. The funding estimates presented are based on adjustments for changes in population and cost-of-living increases since *Best Practices — 2007* was published. The actual funding required for implementing programs will vary depending on state characteristics, such as prevalence of tobacco use, sociodemographic factors, and other factors. See Appendix E for data sources on deaths, costs, revenue, and state-specific factors.

Centers for Disease Control and Prevention • Office on Smoking and Health
www.cdc.gov/tobacco • tobaccoinfo@cdc.gov • 1 (800) CDC-INFO or 1 (800) 232-4636

Section C: Recommended Funding Levels, by State — **Best Practices for Comprehensive Tobacco Control Programs**

Massachusetts

Program Intervention Budgets — 2014

Recommended Annual Investment	$66.9 million
Deaths in State Caused by Smoking	
Annual average smoking-attributable deaths	8,100
Youth aged 0-17 projected to die from smoking	103,100
Annual Costs Incurred in State from Smoking	
Total medical	$4,081 million
State Revenue from Tobacco Sales and Settlement	
FY 2012 tobacco tax revenue	$571.9 million
FY 2012 tobacco settlement payment	$253.6 million
Total state revenue from tobacco sales and settlement	$825.5 million
Percent Tobacco Revenue to Fund at Recommended Level	8%

	Annual Total (Millions)		Annual Per Capita	
	Minimum	Recommended	Minimum	Recommended
I. State and Community Interventions Multiple social resources working together will have the greatest long-term population impact.	$16.9	$21.2	$2.54	$3.19
II. Mass-Reach Health Communication Interventions Media interventions work to prevent smoking initiation, promote cessation, and shape social norms.	$8.9	$12.8	$1.34	$1.93
III. Cessation Interventions Tobacco use treatment is effective and highly cost-effective.	$15.1	$24.2	$2.27	$3.64
IV. Surveillance and Evaluation Publicly funded programs should be accountable and demonstrate effectiveness.	$4.1	$5.8	$0.62	$0.88
V. Infrastructure, Administration, and Management Complex, integrated programs require experienced staff to provide fiscal management, accountability, and coordination.	$2.0	$2.9	$0.31	$0.44
TOTAL	$47.0	$66.9	$7.08	$10.08

Note: A justification for each program element and the rationale for the budget estimates are provided in Section A. The funding estimates presented are based on adjustments for changes in population and cost-of-living increases since *Best Practices — 2007* was published. The actual funding required for implementing programs will vary depending on state characteristics, such as prevalence of tobacco use, sociodemographic factors, and other factors. See Appendix E for data sources on deaths, costs, revenue, and state-specific factors.

Centers for Disease Control and Prevention • Office on Smoking and Health
www.cdc.gov/tobacco • tobaccoinfo@cdc.gov • 1 (800) CDC-INFO or 1 (800) 232-4636

Best Practices for Comprehensive Tobacco Control Programs
Section C: Recommended Funding Levels, by State

Michigan

Program Intervention Budgets — 2014

Recommended Annual Investment	$110.6 million
Deaths in State Caused by Smoking	
Annual average smoking-attributable deaths	14,200
Youth aged 0-17 projected to die from smoking	213,300
Annual Costs Incurred in State from Smoking	
Total medical	$4,590 million
State Revenue from Tobacco Sales and Settlement	
FY 2012 tobacco tax revenue	$972.3 million
FY 2012 tobacco settlement payment	$256.2 million
Total state revenue from tobacco sales and settlement	$1,228.5 million
Percent Tobacco Revenue to Fund at Recommended Level	9%

	Annual Total (Millions)		Annual Per Capita	
	Minimum	Recommended	Minimum	Recommended
I. State and Community Interventions Multiple social resources working together will have the greatest long-term population impact.	$28.3	$35.4	$2.86	$3.58
II. Mass-Reach Health Communication Interventions Media interventions work to prevent smoking initiation, promote cessation, and shape social norms.	$7.9	$11.4	$0.80	$1.15
III. Cessation Interventions Tobacco use treatment is effective and highly cost-effective.	$30.7	$49.4	$3.11	$5.00
IV. Surveillance and Evaluation Publicly funded programs should be accountable and demonstrate effectiveness.	$6.7	$9.6	$0.68	$0.97
V. Infrastructure, Administration, and Management Complex, integrated programs require experienced staff to provide fiscal management, accountability, and coordination.	$3.3	$4.8	$0.34	$0.49
TOTAL	$76.9	$110.6	$7.79	$11.19

Note: A justification for each program element and the rationale for the budget estimates are provided in Section A. The funding estimates presented are based on adjustments for changes in population and cost-of-living increases since *Best Practices—2007* was published. The actual funding required for implementing programs will vary depending on state characteristics, such as prevalence of tobacco use, sociodemographic factors, and other factors. See Appendix E for data sources on deaths, costs, revenue, and state-specific factors.

Centers for Disease Control and Prevention • Office on Smoking and Health
www.cdc.gov/tobacco • tobaccoinfo@cdc.gov • 1 (800) CDC-INFO or 1 (800) 232-4636

Section C: Recommended Funding Levels, by State — Best Practices for Comprehensive Tobacco Control Programs

Minnesota

Program Intervention Budgets — 2014

Recommended Annual Investment	$52.9 million
Deaths in State Caused by Smoking	
Annual average smoking-attributable deaths	5,400
Youth aged 0-17 projected to die from smoking	102,100
Annual Costs Incurred in State from Smoking	
Total medical	$2,519 million
State Revenue from Tobacco Sales and Settlement	
FY 2012 tobacco tax revenue	$375.6 million
FY 2012 tobacco settlement payment	$166.9 million
Total state revenue from tobacco sales and settlement	$542.5 million
Percent Tobacco Revenue to Fund at Recommended Level	10%

	Annual Total (Millions)		Annual Per Capita	
	Minimum	Recommended	Minimum	Recommended
I. State and Community Interventions Multiple social resources working together will have the greatest long-term population impact.	$13.5	$16.8	$2.51	$3.12
II. Mass-Reach Health Communication Interventions Media interventions work to prevent smoking initiation, promote cessation, and shape social norms.	$5.2	$7.5	$0.97	$1.39
III. Cessation Interventions Tobacco use treatment is effective and highly cost-effective.	$13.6	$21.7	$2.53	$4.03
IV. Surveillance and Evaluation Publicly funded programs should be accountable and demonstrate effectiveness.	$3.2	$4.6	$0.60	$0.85
V. Infrastructure, Administration, and Management Complex, integrated programs require experienced staff to provide fiscal management, accountability, and coordination.	$1.6	$2.3	$0.30	$0.43
TOTAL	$37.1	$52.9	$6.91	$9.82

Note: A justification for each program element and the rationale for the budget estimates are provided in Section A. The funding estimates presented are based on adjustments for changes in population and cost-of-living increases since Best Practices — 2007 was published. The actual funding required for implementing programs will vary depending on state characteristics, such as prevalence of tobacco use, sociodemographic factors, and other factors. See Appendix E for data sources on deaths, costs, revenue, and state-specific factors.

Centers for Disease Control and Prevention • Office on Smoking and Health
www.cdc.gov/tobacco • tobaccoinfo@cdc.gov • 1 (800) CDC-INFO or 1 (800) 232-4636

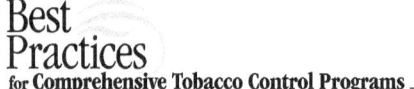

Mississippi

Program Intervention Budgets — 2014

Recommended Annual Investment	**$36.5 million**
Deaths in State Caused by Smoking	
Annual average smoking-attributable deaths	4,700
Youth aged 0-17 projected to die from smoking	68,500
Annual Costs Incurred in State from Smoking	
Total medical	$1,237 million
State Revenue from Tobacco Sales and Settlement	
FY 2012 tobacco tax revenue	$151.6 million
FY 2012 tobacco settlement payment	$113.0 million
Total state revenue from tobacco sales and settlement	$264.6 million
Percent Tobacco Revenue to Fund at Recommended Level	**14%**

	Annual Total (Millions)		Annual Per Capita	
	Minimum	Recommended	Minimum	Recommended
I. State and Community Interventions Multiple social resources working together will have the greatest long-term population impact.	$10.0	$12.5	$3.35	$4.19
II. Mass-Reach Health Communication Interventions Media interventions work to prevent smoking initiation, promote cessation, and shape social norms.	$2.9	$4.1	$0.97	$1.37
III. Cessation Interventions Tobacco use treatment is effective and highly cost-effective.	$9.5	$15.1	$3.18	$5.06
IV. Surveillance and Evaluation Publicly funded programs should be accountable and demonstrate effectiveness.	$2.2	$3.2	$0.75	$1.06
V. Infrastructure, Administration, and Management Complex, integrated programs require experienced staff to provide fiscal management, accountability, and coordination.	$1.1	$1.6	$0.38	$0.53
TOTAL	$25.7	$36.5	$8.63	$12.21

Note: A justification for each program element and the rationale for the budget estimates are provided in Section A. The funding estimates presented are based on adjustments for changes in population and cost-of-living increases since *Best Practices — 2007* was published. The actual funding required for implementing programs will vary depending on state characteristics, such as prevalence of tobacco use, sociodemographic factors, and other factors. See Appendix E for data sources on deaths, costs, revenue, and state-specific factors.

Centers for Disease Control and Prevention • Office on Smoking and Health
www.cdc.gov/tobacco • tobaccoinfo@cdc.gov • 1 (800) CDC-INFO or 1 (800) 232-4636

Section C: Recommended Funding Levels, by State — Best Practices for Comprehensive Tobacco Control Programs

Missouri

Program Intervention Budgets — 2014

Recommended Annual Investment	$72.9 million
Deaths in State Caused by Smoking	
Annual average smoking-attributable deaths	9,600
Youth aged 0-17 projected to die from smoking	127,500
Annual Costs Incurred in State from Smoking	
Total medical	$3,032 million
State Revenue from Tobacco Sales and Settlement	
FY 2012 tobacco tax revenue	$104.9 million
FY 2012 tobacco settlement payment	$135.2 million
Total state revenue from tobacco sales and settlement	$240.1 million
Percent Tobacco Revenue to Fund at Recommended Level	30%

	Annual Total (Millions)		Annual Per Capita	
	Minimum	Recommended	Minimum	Recommended
I. State and Community Interventions Multiple social resources working together will have the greatest long-term population impact.	$17.4	$21.8	$2.89	$3.62
II. Mass-Reach Health Communication Interventions Media interventions work to prevent smoking initiation, promote cessation, and shape social norms.	$7.5	$10.8	$1.25	$1.79
III. Cessation Interventions Tobacco use treatment is effective and highly cost-effective.	$19.2	$30.8	$3.19	$5.11
IV. Surveillance and Evaluation Publicly funded programs should be accountable and demonstrate effectiveness.	$4.4	$6.3	$0.73	$1.05
V. Infrastructure, Administration, and Management Complex, integrated programs require experienced staff to provide fiscal management, accountability, and coordination.	$2.2	$3.2	$0.37	$0.53
TOTAL	$50.7	$72.9	$8.43	$12.10

Note: A justification for each program element and the rationale for the budget estimates are provided in Section A. The funding estimates presented are based on adjustments for changes in population and cost-of-living increases since *Best Practices—2007* was published. The actual funding required for implementing programs will vary depending on state characteristics, such as prevalence of tobacco use, sociodemographic factors, and other factors. See Appendix E for data sources on deaths, costs, revenue, and state-specific factors.

Centers for Disease Control and Prevention • Office on Smoking and Health
www.cdc.gov/tobacco • tobaccoinfo@cdc.gov • 1 (800) CDC-INFO or 1 (800) 232-4636

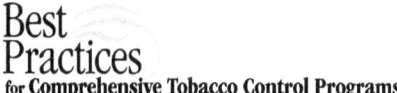

Montana

Program Intervention Budgets — 2014

Recommended Annual Investment	$14.6 million
Deaths in State Caused by Smoking	
Annual average smoking-attributable deaths	1,400
Youth aged 0-17 projected to die from smoking	18,900
Annual Costs Incurred in State from Smoking	
Total medical	$440 million
State Revenue from Tobacco Sales and Settlement	
FY 2012 tobacco tax revenue	$90.0 million
FY 2012 tobacco settlement payment	$30.2 million
Total state revenue from tobacco sales and settlement	$120.2 million
Percent Tobacco Revenue to Fund at Recommended Level	**12%**

	Annual Total (Millions)		Annual Per Capita	
	Minimum	Recommended	Minimum	Recommended
I. State and Community Interventions Multiple social resources working together will have the greatest long-term population impact.	$4.0	$5.0	$3.98	$4.97
II. Mass-Reach Health Communication Interventions Media interventions work to prevent smoking initiation, promote cessation, and shape social norms.	$2.2	$3.1	$2.19	$3.08
III. Cessation Interventions Tobacco use treatment is effective and highly cost-effective.	$2.9	$4.6	$2.89	$4.58
IV. Surveillance and Evaluation Publicly funded programs should be accountable and demonstrate effectiveness.	$0.9	$1.3	$0.91	$1.26
V. Infrastructure, Administration, and Management Complex, integrated programs require experienced staff to provide fiscal management, accountability, and coordination.	$0.5	$0.6	$0.45	$0.63
TOTAL	$10.5	$14.6	$10.42	$14.52

Note: A justification for each program element and the rationale for the budget estimates are provided in Section A. The funding estimates presented are based on adjustments for changes in population and cost-of-living increases since *Best Practices — 2007* was published. The actual funding required for implementing programs will vary depending on state characteristics, such as prevalence of tobacco use, sociodemographic factors, and other factors. See Appendix E for data sources on deaths, costs, revenue, and state-specific factors.

Centers for Disease Control and Prevention • Office on Smoking and Health
www.cdc.gov/tobacco • tobaccoinfo@cdc.gov • 1 (800) CDC-INFO or 1 (800) 232-4636

Section C: Recommended Funding Levels, by State — **Best Practices for Comprehensive Tobacco Control Programs**

Nebraska

Program Intervention Budgets — 2014

Recommended Annual Investment	$20.8 million
Deaths in State Caused by Smoking	
Annual average smoking-attributable deaths	2,200
Youth aged 0-17 projected to die from smoking	38,000
Annual Costs Incurred in State from Smoking	
Total medical	$795 million
State Revenue from Tobacco Sales and Settlement	
FY 2012 tobacco tax revenue	$69.0 million
FY 2012 tobacco settlement payment	$37.7 million
Total state revenue from tobacco sales and settlement	$106.7 million
Percent Tobacco Revenue to Fund at Recommended Level	19%

	Annual Total (Millions)		Annual Per Capita	
	Minimum	Recommended	Minimum	Recommended
I. State and Community Interventions Multiple social resources working together will have the greatest long-term population impact.	$5.3	$6.6	$2.86	$3.56
II. Mass-Reach Health Communication Interventions Media interventions work to prevent smoking initiation, promote cessation, and shape social norms.	$2.5	$3.6	$1.35	$1.94
III. Cessation Interventions Tobacco use treatment is effective and highly cost-effective.	$5.0	$7.9	$2.69	$4.26
IV. Surveillance and Evaluation Publicly funded programs should be accountable and demonstrate effectiveness.	$1.3	$1.8	$0.69	$0.98
V. Infrastructure, Administration, and Management Complex, integrated programs require experienced staff to provide fiscal management, accountability, and coordination.	$0.6	$0.9	$0.35	$0.49
TOTAL	$14.7	$20.8	$7.94	$11.23

Note: A justification for each program element and the rationale for the budget estimates are provided in Section A. The funding estimates presented are based on adjustments for changes in population and cost-of-living increases since *Best Practices—2007* was published. The actual funding required for implementing programs will vary depending on state characteristics, such as prevalence of tobacco use, sociodemographic factors, and other factors. See Appendix E for data sources on deaths, costs, revenue, and state-specific factors.

Centers for Disease Control and Prevention • Office on Smoking and Health
www.cdc.gov/tobacco • tobaccoinfo@cdc.gov • 1 (800) CDC-INFO or 1 (800) 232-4636

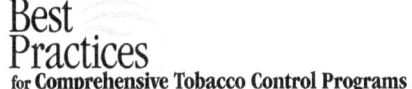

Nevada

Program Intervention Budgets — 2014

Recommended Annual Investment	**$30.0 million**
Deaths in State Caused by Smoking	
Annual average smoking-attributable deaths	3,500
Youth aged 0-17 projected to die from smoking	41,200
Annual Costs Incurred in State from Smoking	
Total medical	$1,080 million
State Revenue from Tobacco Sales and Settlement	
FY 2012 tobacco tax revenue	$102.4 million
FY 2012 tobacco settlement payment	$40.3 million
Total state revenue from tobacco sales and settlement	$142.7 million
Percent Tobacco Revenue to Fund at Recommended Level	**21%**

	Annual Total (Millions)		Annual Per Capita	
	Minimum	Recommended	Minimum	Recommended
I. State and Community Interventions Multiple social resources working together will have the greatest long-term population impact.	$8.3	$10.4	$3.01	$3.77
II. Mass-Reach Health Communication Interventions Media interventions work to prevent smoking initiation, promote cessation, and shape social norms.	$3.4	$4.9	$1.23	$1.78
III. Cessation Interventions Tobacco use treatment is effective and highly cost-effective.	$6.8	$10.8	$2.46	$3.91
IV. Surveillance and Evaluation Publicly funded programs should be accountable and demonstrate effectiveness.	$1.9	$2.6	$0.67	$0.95
V. Infrastructure, Administration, and Management Complex, integrated programs require experienced staff to provide fiscal management, accountability, and coordination.	$0.9	$1.3	$0.34	$0.47
TOTAL	$21.3	$30.0	$7.71	$10.88

Note: A justification for each program element and the rationale for the budget estimates are provided in Section A. The funding estimates presented are based on adjustments for changes in population and cost-of-living increases since *Best Practices—2007* was published. The actual funding required for implementing programs will vary depending on state characteristics, such as prevalence of tobacco use, sociodemographic factors, and other factors. See Appendix E for data sources on deaths, costs, revenue, and state-specific factors.

Section C: Recommended Funding Levels, by State — **Best Practices for Comprehensive Tobacco Control Programs**

New Hampshire

Program Intervention Budgets — 2014

Recommended Annual Investment	**$16.5 million**
Deaths in State Caused by Smoking	
Annual average smoking-attributable deaths	1,700
Youth aged 0-17 projected to die from smoking	21,700
Annual Costs Incurred in State from Smoking	
Total medical	$729 million
State Revenue from Tobacco Sales and Settlement	
FY 2012 tobacco tax revenue	$215.1 million
FY 2012 tobacco settlement payment	$42.5 million
Total state revenue from tobacco sales and settlement	$257.6 million
Percent Tobacco Revenue to Fund at Recommended Level	6%

	Annual Total (Millions)		Annual Per Capita	
	Minimum	**Recommended**	**Minimum**	**Recommended**
I. State and Community Interventions Multiple social resources working together will have the greatest long-term population impact.	$4.0	$5.0	$3.03	$3.79
II. Mass-Reach Health Communication Interventions Media interventions work to prevent smoking initiation, promote cessation, and shape social norms.	$2.8	$4.1	$2.12	$3.10
III. Cessation Interventions Tobacco use treatment is effective and highly cost-effective.	$3.4	$5.3	$2.57	$4.01
IV. Surveillance and Evaluation Publicly funded programs should be accountable and demonstrate effectiveness.	$1.0	$1.4	$0.77	$1.09
V. Infrastructure, Administration, and Management Complex, integrated programs require experienced staff to provide fiscal management, accountability, and coordination.	$0.5	$0.7	$0.39	$0.55
TOTAL	$11.7	$16.5	$8.88	$12.54

Note: A justification for each program element and the rationale for the budget estimates are provided in Section A. The funding estimates presented are based on adjustments for changes in population and cost-of-living increases since *Best Practices — 2007* was published. The actual funding required for implementing programs will vary depending on state characteristics, such as prevalence of tobacco use, sociodemographic factors, and other factors. See Appendix E for data sources on deaths, costs, revenue, and state-specific factors.

Centers for Disease Control and Prevention • Office on Smoking and Health
www.cdc.gov/tobacco • tobaccoinfo@cdc.gov • 1 (800) CDC-INFO or 1 (800) 232-4636

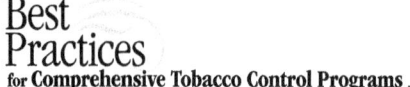

Section C: Recommended Funding Levels, by State

New Jersey

Program Intervention Budgets — 2014

Recommended Annual Investment	$103.3 million
Deaths in State Caused by Smoking	
Annual average smoking-attributable deaths	10,100
Youth aged 0-17 projected to die from smoking	142,700
Annual Costs Incurred in State from Smoking	
Total medical	$4,066 million
State Revenue from Tobacco Sales and Settlement	
FY 2012 tobacco tax revenue	$772.8 million
FY 2012 tobacco settlement payment	$231.3 million
Total state revenue from tobacco sales and settlement	$1,004.1 million
Percent Tobacco Revenue to Fund at Recommended Level	**10%**

	Annual Total (Millions)		Annual Per Capita	
	Minimum	Recommended	Minimum	Recommended
I. State and Community Interventions Multiple social resources working together will have the greatest long-term population impact.	$23.4	$29.2	$2.64	$3.29
II. Mass-Reach Health Communication Interventions Media interventions work to prevent smoking initiation, promote cessation, and shape social norms.	$19.1	$27.5	$2.15	$3.10
III. Cessation Interventions Tobacco use treatment is effective and highly cost-effective.	$20.7	$33.1	$2.34	$3.73
IV. Surveillance and Evaluation Publicly funded programs should be accountable and demonstrate effectiveness.	$6.3	$9.0	$0.71	$1.01
V. Infrastructure, Administration, and Management Complex, integrated programs require experienced staff to provide fiscal management, accountability, and coordination.	$3.2	$4.5	$0.36	$0.51
TOTAL	$72.7	$103.3	$8.20	$11.64

Note: A justification for each program element and the rationale for the budget estimates are provided in Section A. The funding estimates presented are based on adjustments for changes in population and cost-of-living increases since *Best Practices — 2007* was published. The actual funding required for implementing programs will vary depending on state characteristics, such as prevalence of tobacco use, sociodemographic factors, and other factors. See Appendix E for data sources on deaths, costs, revenue, and state-specific factors.

Centers for Disease Control and Prevention • Office on Smoking and Health
www.cdc.gov/tobacco • tobaccoinfo@cdc.gov • 1 (800) CDC-INFO or 1 (800) 232-4636

Section C: Recommended Funding Levels, by State — **Best Practices for Comprehensive Tobacco Control Programs**

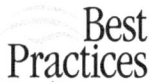

New Mexico

Program Intervention Budgets — 2014

Recommended Annual Investment	$22.8 million
Deaths in State Caused by Smoking	
Annual average smoking-attributable deaths	2,200
Youth aged 0-17 projected to die from smoking	39,800
Annual Costs Incurred in State from Smoking	
Total medical	$844 million
State Revenue from Tobacco Sales and Settlement	
FY 2012 tobacco tax revenue	$99.4 million
FY 2012 tobacco settlement payment	$39.3 million
Total state revenue from tobacco sales and settlement	$138.7 million
Percent Tobacco Revenue to Fund at Recommended Level	16%

	Annual Total (Millions)		Annual Per Capita	
	Minimum	Recommended	Minimum	Recommended
I. State and Community Interventions Multiple social resources working together will have the greatest long-term population impact.	$7.4	$9.3	$3.55	$4.46
II. Mass-Reach Health Communication Interventions Media interventions work to prevent smoking initiation, promote cessation, and shape social norms.	$1.3	$1.8	$0.62	$0.86
III. Cessation Interventions Tobacco use treatment is effective and highly cost-effective.	$5.5	$8.7	$2.64	$4.17
IV. Surveillance and Evaluation Publicly funded programs should be accountable and demonstrate effectiveness.	$1.4	$2.0	$0.68	$0.95
V. Infrastructure, Administration, and Management Complex, integrated programs require experienced staff to provide fiscal management, accountability, and coordination.	$0.7	$1.0	$0.34	$0.47
TOTAL	$16.3	$22.8	$7.83	$10.91

Note: A justification for each program element and the rationale for the budget estimates are provided in Section A. The funding estimates presented are based on adjustments for changes in population and cost-of-living increases since *Best Practices—2007* was published. The actual funding required for implementing programs will vary depending on state characteristics, such as prevalence of tobacco use, sociodemographic factors, and other factors. See Appendix E for data sources on deaths, costs, revenue, and state-specific factors.

Centers for Disease Control and Prevention • Office on Smoking and Health
www.cdc.gov/tobacco • tobaccoinfo@cdc.gov • 1 (800) CDC-INFO or 1 (800) 232-4636

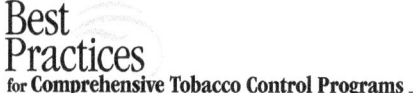

Section C: Recommended Funding Levels, by State

New York

Program Intervention Budgets — 2014

Recommended Annual Investment	$203.0 million
Deaths in State Caused by Smoking	
Annual average smoking-attributable deaths	23,600
Youth aged 0-17 projected to die from smoking	279,700
Annual Costs Incurred in State from Smoking	
Total medical	$10,390 million
State Revenue from Tobacco Sales and Settlement	
FY 2012 tobacco tax revenue	$1,630.5 million
FY 2012 tobacco settlement payment	$737.7 million
Total state revenue from tobacco sales and settlement	$2,368.2 million
Percent Tobacco Revenue to Fund at Recommended Level	9%

	Annual Total (Millions)		Annual Per Capita	
	Minimum	Recommended	Minimum	Recommended
I. State and Community Interventions Multiple social resources working together will have the greatest long-term population impact.	$49.3	$61.6	$2.52	$3.15
II. Mass-Reach Health Communication Interventions Media interventions work to prevent smoking initiation, promote cessation, and shape social norms.	$31.8	$45.7	$1.62	$2.34
III. Cessation Interventions Tobacco use treatment is effective and highly cost-effective.	$43.1	$69.2	$2.20	$3.54
IV. Surveillance and Evaluation Publicly funded programs should be accountable and demonstrate effectiveness.	$12.4	$17.7	$0.63	$0.90
V. Infrastructure, Administration, and Management Complex, integrated programs require experienced staff to provide fiscal management, accountability, and coordination.	$6.2	$8.8	$0.32	$0.45
TOTAL	$142.8	$203.0	$7.29	$10.38

Note: A justification for each program element and the rationale for the budget estimates are provided in Section A. The funding estimates presented are based on adjustments for changes in population and cost-of-living increases since *Best Practices — 2007* was published. The actual funding required for implementing programs will vary depending on state characteristics, such as prevalence of tobacco use, sociodemographic factors, and other factors. See Appendix E for data sources on deaths, costs, revenue, and state-specific factors.

Centers for Disease Control and Prevention • Office on Smoking and Health
www.cdc.gov/tobacco • tobaccoinfo@cdc.gov • 1 (800) CDC-INFO or 1 (800) 232-4636

Section C: Recommended Funding Levels, by State — 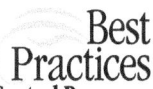 **Best Practices** for **Comprehensive Tobacco Control Programs**

North Carolina

Program Intervention Budgets — 2014

Recommended Annual Investment	**$99.3 million**
Deaths in State Caused by Smoking	
Annual average smoking-attributable deaths	12,500
Youth aged 0-17 projected to die from smoking	180,000
Annual Costs Incurred in State from Smoking	
Total medical	$3,810 million
State Revenue from Tobacco Sales and Settlement	
FY 2012 tobacco tax revenue	$294.8 million
FY 2012 tobacco settlement payment	$141.0 million
Total state revenue from tobacco sales and settlement	$435.8 million
Percent Tobacco Revenue to Fund at Recommended Level	23%

	Annual Total (Millions)		Annual Per Capita	
	Minimum	Recommended	Minimum	Recommended
I. State and Community Interventions Multiple social resources working together will have the greatest long-term population impact.	$26.4	$33.1	$2.71	$3.39
II. Mass-Reach Health Communication Interventions Media interventions work to prevent smoking initiation, promote cessation, and shape social norms.	$6.8	$9.8	$0.70	$1.00
III. Cessation Interventions Tobacco use treatment is effective and highly cost-effective.	$27.1	$43.5	$2.78	$4.46
IV. Surveillance and Evaluation Publicly funded programs should be accountable and demonstrate effectiveness.	$6.0	$8.6	$0.62	$0.89
V. Infrastructure, Administration, and Management Complex, integrated programs require experienced staff to provide fiscal management, accountability, and coordination.	$3.0	$4.3	$0.31	$0.44
TOTAL	$69.3	$99.3	$7.12	$10.18

Note: A justification for each program element and the rationale for the budget estimates are provided in Section A. The funding estimates presented are based on adjustments for changes in population and cost-of-living increases since *Best Practices — 2007* was published. The actual funding required for implementing programs will vary depending on state characteristics, such as prevalence of tobacco use, sociodemographic factors, and other factors. See Appendix E for data sources on deaths, costs, revenue, and state-specific factors.

Centers for Disease Control and Prevention • Office on Smoking and Health
www.cdc.gov/tobacco • tobaccoinfo@cdc.gov • 1 (800) CDC-INFO or 1 (800) 232-4636

North Dakota

Program Intervention Budgets — 2014

Recommended Annual Investment	**$9.8 million**
Deaths in State Caused by Smoking	
Annual average smoking-attributable deaths	800
Youth aged 0-17 projected to die from smoking	13,900
Annual Costs Incurred in State from Smoking	
Total medical	$326 million
State Revenue from Tobacco Sales and Settlement	
FY 2012 tobacco tax revenue	$28.2 million
FY 2012 tobacco settlement payment	$31.5 million
Total state revenue from tobacco sales and settlement	$59.7 million
Percent Tobacco Revenue to Fund at Recommended Level	**16%**

	Annual Total (Millions)		Annual Per Capita	
	Minimum	Recommended	Minimum	Recommended
I. State and Community Interventions Multiple social resources working together will have the greatest long-term population impact.	$2.9	$3.7	$4.15	$5.29
II. Mass-Reach Health Communication Interventions Media interventions work to prevent smoking initiation, promote cessation, and shape social norms.	$0.9	$1.3	$1.29	$1.86
III. Cessation Interventions Tobacco use treatment is effective and highly cost-effective.	$2.3	$3.5	$3.29	$5.00
IV. Surveillance and Evaluation Publicly funded programs should be accountable and demonstrate effectiveness.	$0.6	$0.9	$0.87	$1.22
V. Infrastructure, Administration, and Management Complex, integrated programs require experienced staff to provide fiscal management, accountability, and coordination.	$0.3	$0.4	$0.44	$0.61
TOTAL	$7.0	$9.8	$10.04	$13.98

Note: A justification for each program element and the rationale for the budget estimates are provided in Section A. The funding estimates presented are based on adjustments for changes in population and cost-of-living increases since *Best Practices — 2007* was published. The actual funding required for implementing programs will vary depending on state characteristics, such as prevalence of tobacco use, sociodemographic factors, and other factors. See Appendix E for data sources on deaths, costs, revenue, and state-specific factors.

Section C: Recommended Funding Levels, by State — Best Practices for Comprehensive Tobacco Control Programs

Ohio

Program Intervention Budgets — 2014

Recommended Annual Investment	**$132.0 million**
Deaths in State Caused by Smoking	
Annual average smoking-attributable deaths	17,700
Youth aged 0-17 projected to die from smoking	259,100
Annual Costs Incurred in State from Smoking	
Total medical	$5,647 million
State Revenue from Tobacco Sales and Settlement	
FY 2012 tobacco tax revenue	$841.8 million
FY 2012 tobacco settlement payment	$295.2 million
Total state revenue from tobacco sales and settlement	$1,137.0 million
Percent Tobacco Revenue to Fund at Recommended Level	**12%**

	Annual Total (Millions)		Annual Per Capita	
	Minimum	Recommended	Minimum	Recommended
I. State and Community Interventions Multiple social resources working together will have the greatest long-term population impact.	$34.3	$42.9	$2.97	$3.72
II. Mass-Reach Health Communication Interventions Media interventions work to prevent smoking initiation, promote cessation, and shape social norms.	$10.0	$14.4	$0.87	$1.25
III. Cessation Interventions Tobacco use treatment is effective and highly cost-effective.	$35.7	$57.5	$3.09	$4.98
IV. Surveillance and Evaluation Publicly funded programs should be accountable and demonstrate effectiveness.	$8.0	$11.5	$0.69	$1.00
V. Infrastructure, Administration, and Management Complex, integrated programs require experienced staff to provide fiscal management, accountability, and coordination.	$4.0	$5.7	$0.35	$0.50
TOTAL	$92.0	$132.0	$7.97	$11.45

Note: A justification for each program element and the rationale for the budget estimates are provided in Section A. The funding estimates presented are based on adjustments for changes in population and cost-of-living increases since Best Practices—2007 was published. The actual funding required for implementing programs will vary depending on state characteristics, such as prevalence of tobacco use, sociodemographic factors, and other factors. See Appendix E for data sources on deaths, costs, revenue, and state-specific factors.

Centers for Disease Control and Prevention • Office on Smoking and Health
www.cdc.gov/tobacco • tobaccoinfo@cdc.gov • 1 (800) CDC-INFO or 1 (800) 232-4636

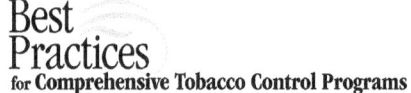

Oklahoma

Program Intervention Budgets — 2014

Recommended Annual Investment	**$42.3 million**
Deaths in State Caused by Smoking	
Annual average smoking-attributable deaths	6,500
Youth aged 0-17 projected to die from smoking	88,200
Annual Costs Incurred in State from Smoking	
Total medical	$1,622 million
State Revenue from Tobacco Sales and Settlement	
FY 2012 tobacco tax revenue	$291.3 million
FY 2012 tobacco settlement payment	$77.4 million
Total state revenue from tobacco sales and settlement	$368.7 million
Percent Tobacco Revenue to Fund at Recommended Level	**11%**

	Annual Total (Millions)		Annual Per Capita	
	Minimum	Recommended	Minimum	Recommended
I. State and Community Interventions Multiple social resources working together will have the greatest long-term population impact.	$11.7	$14.6	$3.07	$3.83
II. Mass-Reach Health Communication Interventions Media interventions work to prevent smoking initiation, promote cessation, and shape social norms.	$2.4	$3.4	$0.63	$0.89
III. Cessation Interventions Tobacco use treatment is effective and highly cost-effective.	$11.8	$18.8	$3.09	$4.93
IV. Surveillance and Evaluation Publicly funded programs should be accountable and demonstrate effectiveness.	$2.6	$3.7	$0.68	$0.97
V. Infrastructure, Administration, and Management Complex, integrated programs require experienced staff to provide fiscal management, accountability, and coordination.	$1.3	$1.8	$0.34	$0.48
TOTAL	$29.8	$42.3	$7.81	$11.10

Note: A justification for each program element and the rationale for the budget estimates are provided in Section A. The funding estimates presented are based on adjustments for changes in population and cost-of-living increases since *Best Practices — 2007* was published. The actual funding required for implementing programs will vary depending on state characteristics, such as prevalence of tobacco use, sociodemographic factors, and other factors. See Appendix E for data sources on deaths, costs, revenue, and state-specific factors.

Centers for Disease Control and Prevention • Office on Smoking and Health
www.cdc.gov/tobacco • tobaccoinfo@cdc.gov • 1 (800) CDC-INFO or 1 (800) 232-4636

Section C: Recommended Funding Levels, by State — **Best Practices for Comprehensive Tobacco Control Programs**

Oregon

Program Intervention Budgets — 2014

Recommended Annual Investment	$39.3 million
Deaths in State Caused by Smoking	
Annual average smoking-attributable deaths	4,800
Youth aged 0-17 projected to die from smoking	68,300
Annual Costs Incurred in State from Smoking	
Total medical	$1,548 million
State Revenue from Tobacco Sales and Settlement	
FY 2012 tobacco tax revenue	$255.7 million
FY 2012 tobacco settlement payment	$78.9 million
Total state revenue from tobacco sales and settlement	$334.6 million
Percent Tobacco Revenue to Fund at Recommended Level	12%

	Annual Total (Millions)		Annual Per Capita	
	Minimum	Recommended	Minimum	Recommended
I. State and Community Interventions Multiple social resources working together will have the greatest long-term population impact.	$10.3	$12.9	$2.64	$3.31
II. Mass-Reach Health Communication Interventions Media interventions work to prevent smoking initiation, promote cessation, and shape social norms.	$4.1	$5.9	$1.05	$1.51
III. Cessation Interventions Tobacco use treatment is effective and highly cost-effective.	$9.7	$15.4	$2.49	$3.95
IV. Surveillance and Evaluation Publicly funded programs should be accountable and demonstrate effectiveness.	$2.4	$3.4	$0.62	$0.88
V. Infrastructure, Administration, and Management Complex, integrated programs require experienced staff to provide fiscal management, accountability, and coordination.	$1.2	$1.7	$0.31	$0.44
TOTAL	$27.7	$39.3	$7.11	$10.09

Note: A justification for each program element and the rationale for the budget estimates are provided in Section A. The funding estimates presented are based on adjustments for changes in population and cost-of-living increases since *Best Practices — 2007* was published. The actual funding required for implementing programs will vary depending on state characteristics, such as prevalence of tobacco use, sociodemographic factors, and other factors. See Appendix E for data sources on deaths, costs, revenue, and state-specific factors.

Centers for Disease Control and Prevention • Office on Smoking and Health
www.cdc.gov/tobacco • tobaccoinfo@cdc.gov • 1 (800) CDC-INFO or 1 (800) 232-4636

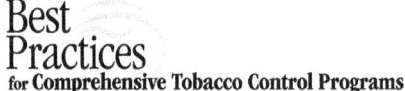

Pennsylvania

Program Intervention Budgets — 2014

Recommended Annual Investment	$140.0 million
Deaths in State Caused by Smoking	
Annual average smoking-attributable deaths	19,200
Youth aged 0-17 projected to die from smoking	243,700
Annual Costs Incurred in State from Smoking	
Total medical	$6,383 million
State Revenue from Tobacco Sales and Settlement	
FY 2012 tobacco tax revenue	$1,116.7 million
FY 2012 tobacco settlement payment	$337.4 million
Total state revenue from tobacco sales and settlement	$1,454.1 million
Percent Tobacco Revenue to Fund at Recommended Level	**10%**

	Annual Total (Millions)		Annual Per Capita	
	Minimum	Recommended	Minimum	Recommended
I. State and Community Interventions Multiple social resources working together will have the greatest long-term population impact.	$32.7	$40.8	$2.56	$3.20
II. Mass-Reach Health Communication Interventions Media interventions work to prevent smoking initiation, promote cessation, and shape social norms.	$14.8	$21.3	$1.16	$1.67
III. Cessation Interventions Tobacco use treatment is effective and highly cost-effective.	$37.1	$59.6	$2.91	$4.67
IV. Surveillance and Evaluation Publicly funded programs should be accountable and demonstrate effectiveness.	$8.5	$12.2	$0.66	$0.95
V. Infrastructure, Administration, and Management Complex, integrated programs require experienced staff to provide fiscal management, accountability, and coordination.	$4.2	$6.1	$0.33	$0.48
TOTAL	$97.3	$140.0	$7.62	$10.97

Note: A justification for each program element and the rationale for the budget estimates are provided in Section A. The funding estimates presented are based on adjustments for changes in population and cost-of-living increases since *Best Practices—2007* was published. The actual funding required for implementing programs will vary depending on state characteristics, such as prevalence of tobacco use, sociodemographic factors, and other factors. See Appendix E for data sources on deaths, costs, revenue, and state-specific factors.

Section C: Recommended Funding Levels, by State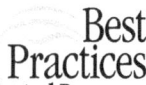

Rhode Island

Program Intervention Budgets — 2014

Recommended Annual Investment	$12.8 million
Deaths in State Caused by Smoking	
Annual average smoking-attributable deaths	1,500
Youth aged 0-17 projected to die from smoking	15,600
Annual Costs Incurred in State from Smoking	
Total medical	$640 million
State Revenue from Tobacco Sales and Settlement	
FY 2012 tobacco tax revenue	$132.1 million
FY 2012 tobacco settlement payment	$46.7 million
Total state revenue from tobacco sales and settlement	$178.8 million
Percent Tobacco Revenue to Fund at Recommended Level	7%

	Annual Total (Millions)		Annual Per Capita	
	Minimum	Recommended	Minimum	Recommended
I. State and Community Interventions Multiple social resources working together will have the greatest long-term population impact.	$3.8	$4.7	$3.62	$4.47
II. Mass-Reach Health Communication Interventions Media interventions work to prevent smoking initiation, promote cessation, and shape social norms.	$1.5	$2.1	$1.43	$2.00
III. Cessation Interventions Tobacco use treatment is effective and highly cost-effective.	$2.8	$4.3	$2.67	$4.09
IV. Surveillance and Evaluation Publicly funded programs should be accountable and demonstrate effectiveness.	$0.8	$1.1	$0.77	$1.06
V. Infrastructure, Administration, and Management Complex, integrated programs require experienced staff to provide fiscal management, accountability, and coordination.	$0.4	$0.6	$0.39	$0.53
TOTAL	$9.3	$12.8	$8.88	$12.15

Note: A justification for each program element and the rationale for the budget estimates are provided in Section A. The funding estimates presented are based on adjustments for changes in population and cost-of-living increases since *Best Practices — 2007* was published. The actual funding required for implementing programs will vary depending on state characteristics, such as prevalence of tobacco use, sociodemographic factors, and other factors. See Appendix E for data sources on deaths, costs, revenue, and state-specific factors.

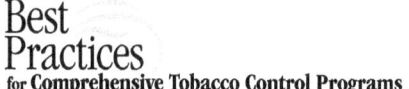

South Carolina

Program Intervention Budgets — 2014

Recommended Annual Investment	$51.0 million
Deaths in State Caused by Smoking	
Annual average smoking-attributable deaths	6,400
Youth aged 0-17 projected to die from smoking	103,300
Annual Costs Incurred in State from Smoking	
Total medical	$1,907 million
State Revenue from Tobacco Sales and Settlement	
FY 2012 tobacco tax revenue	$165.7 million
FY 2012 tobacco settlement payment	$73.4 million
Total state revenue from tobacco sales and settlement	$239.1 million
Percent Tobacco Revenue to Fund at Recommended Level	**21%**

	Annual Total (Millions)		Annual Per Capita	
	Minimum	Recommended	Minimum	Recommended
I. State and Community Interventions Multiple social resources working together will have the greatest long-term population impact.	$13.4	$16.7	$2.84	$3.54
II. Mass-Reach Health Communication Interventions Media interventions work to prevent smoking initiation, promote cessation, and shape social norms.	$3.2	$4.7	$0.68	$0.99
III. Cessation Interventions Tobacco use treatment is effective and highly cost-effective.	$14.3	$23.0	$3.03	$4.87
IV. Surveillance and Evaluation Publicly funded programs should be accountable and demonstrate effectiveness.	$3.1	$4.4	$0.66	$0.94
V. Infrastructure, Administration, and Management Complex, integrated programs require experienced staff to provide fiscal management, accountability, and coordination.	$1.5	$2.2	$0.33	$0.47
TOTAL	$35.5	$51.0	$7.54	$10.81

Note: A justification for each program element and the rationale for the budget estimates are provided in Section A. The funding estimates presented are based on adjustments for changes in population and cost-of-living increases since Best Practices—2007 was published. The actual funding required for implementing programs will vary depending on state characteristics, such as prevalence of tobacco use, sociodemographic factors, and other factors. See Appendix E for data sources on deaths, costs, revenue, and state-specific factors.

Section C: Recommended Funding Levels, by State — **Best Practices** for Comprehensive Tobacco Control Programs

South Dakota

Program Intervention Budgets — 2014

Recommended Annual Investment	**$11.7 million**
Deaths in State Caused by Smoking	
Annual average smoking-attributable deaths	1,100
Youth aged 0-17 projected to die from smoking	21,000
Annual Costs Incurred in State from Smoking	
Total medical	$373 million
State Revenue from Tobacco Sales and Settlement	
FY 2012 tobacco tax revenue	$60.1 million
FY 2012 tobacco settlement payment	$24.1 million
Total state revenue from tobacco sales and settlement	$84.2 million
Percent Tobacco Revenue to Fund at Recommended Level	**14%**

	Annual Total (Millions)		Annual Per Capita	
	Minimum	Recommended	Minimum	Recommended
I. State and Community Interventions Multiple social resources working together will have the greatest long-term population impact.	$3.5	$4.4	$4.20	$5.28
II. Mass-Reach Health Communication Interventions Media interventions work to prevent smoking initiation, promote cessation, and shape social norms.	$1.2	$1.7	$1.44	$2.04
III. Cessation Interventions Tobacco use treatment is effective and highly cost-effective.	$2.7	$4.1	$3.24	$4.92
IV. Surveillance and Evaluation Publicly funded programs should be accountable and demonstrate effectiveness.	$0.7	$1.0	$0.89	$1.22
V. Infrastructure, Administration, and Management Complex, integrated programs require experienced staff to provide fiscal management, accountability, and coordination.	$0.4	$0.5	$0.44	$0.61
TOTAL	$8.5	$11.7	$10.21	$14.07

Note: A justification for each program element and the rationale for the budget estimates are provided in Section A. The funding estimates presented are based on adjustments for changes in population and cost-of-living increases since *Best Practices — 2007* was published. The actual funding required for implementing programs will vary depending on state characteristics, such as prevalence of tobacco use, sociodemographic factors, and other factors. See Appendix E for data sources on deaths, costs, revenue, and state-specific factors.

Centers for Disease Control and Prevention • Office on Smoking and Health
www.cdc.gov/tobacco • tobaccoinfo@cdc.gov • 1 (800) CDC-INFO or 1 (800) 232-4636

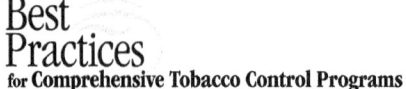
Section C: Recommended Funding Levels, by State

Tennessee

Program Intervention Budgets — 2014

Recommended Annual Investment	$75.6 million
Deaths in State Caused by Smoking	
Annual average smoking-attributable deaths	10,000
Youth aged 0-17 projected to die from smoking	125,300
Annual Costs Incurred in State from Smoking	
Total medical	$2,673 million
State Revenue from Tobacco Sales and Settlement	
FY 2012 tobacco tax revenue	$278.6 million
FY 2012 tobacco settlement payment	$139.2 million
Total state revenue from tobacco sales and settlement	$417.8 million
Percent Tobacco Revenue to Fund at Recommended Level	**18%**

	Annual Total (Millions)		Annual Per Capita	
	Minimum	Recommended	Minimum	Recommended
I. State and Community Interventions Multiple social resources working together will have the greatest long-term population impact.	$18.7	$23.4	$2.90	$3.62
II. Mass-Reach Health Communication Interventions Media interventions work to prevent smoking initiation, promote cessation, and shape social norms.	$5.5	$7.9	$0.85	$1.22
III. Cessation Interventions Tobacco use treatment is effective and highly cost-effective.	$21.4	$34.4	$3.31	$5.33
IV. Surveillance and Evaluation Publicly funded programs should be accountable and demonstrate effectiveness.	$4.6	$6.6	$0.71	$1.02
V. Infrastructure, Administration, and Management Complex, integrated programs require experienced staff to provide fiscal management, accountability, and coordination.	$2.3	$3.3	$0.35	$0.51
TOTAL	$52.5	$75.6	$8.12	$11.70

Note: A justification for each program element and the rationale for the budget estimates are provided in Section A. The funding estimates presented are based on adjustments for changes in population and cost-of-living increases since *Best Practices — 2007* was published. The actual funding required for implementing programs will vary depending on state characteristics, such as prevalence of tobacco use, sociodemographic factors, and other factors. See Appendix E for data sources on deaths, costs, revenue, and state-specific factors.

Centers for Disease Control and Prevention • Office on Smoking and Health
www.cdc.gov/tobacco • tobaccoinfo@cdc.gov • 1 (800) CDC-INFO or 1 (800) 232-4636

Section C: Recommended Funding Levels, by State — **Best Practices** for Comprehensive Tobacco Control Programs

Texas

Program Intervention Budgets — 2014

Recommended Annual Investment	**$264.1 million**
Deaths in State Caused by Smoking	
Annual average smoking-attributable deaths	23,900
Youth aged 0-17 projected to die from smoking	498,500
Annual Costs Incurred in State from Smoking	
Total medical	$8,856 million
State Revenue from Tobacco Sales and Settlement	
FY 2012 tobacco tax revenue	$1,484.0 million
FY 2012 tobacco settlement payment	$474.6 million
Total state revenue from tobacco sales and settlement	$1,958.6 million
Percent Tobacco Revenue to Fund at Recommended Level	**13%**

	Annual Total (Millions)		Annual Per Capita	
	Minimum	Recommended	Minimum	Recommended
I. State and Community Interventions Multiple social resources working together will have the greatest long-term population impact.	$68.0	$85.0	$2.61	$3.26
II. Mass-Reach Health Communication Interventions Media interventions work to prevent smoking initiation, promote cessation, and shape social norms.	$33.3	$47.9	$1.28	$1.84
III. Cessation Interventions Tobacco use treatment is effective and highly cost-effective.	$60.2	$96.7	$2.31	$3.71
IV. Surveillance and Evaluation Publicly funded programs should be accountable and demonstrate effectiveness.	$16.2	$23.0	$0.62	$0.88
V. Infrastructure, Administration, and Management Complex, integrated programs require experienced staff to provide fiscal management, accountability, and coordination.	$8.1	$11.5	$0.31	$0.44
TOTAL	$185.8	$264.1	$7.13	$10.13

Note: A justification for each program element and the rationale for the budget estimates are provided in Section A. The funding estimates presented are based on adjustments for changes in population and cost-of-living increases since *Best Practices — 2007* was published. The actual funding required for implementing programs will vary depending on state characteristics, such as prevalence of tobacco use, sociodemographic factors, and other factors. See Appendix E for data sources on deaths, costs, revenue, and state-specific factors.

Centers for Disease Control and Prevention • Office on Smoking and Health
www.cdc.gov/tobacco • tobaccoinfo@cdc.gov • 1 (800) CDC-INFO or 1 (800) 232-4636

Best Practices for Comprehensive Tobacco Control Programs — *Section C: Recommended Funding Levels, by State*

Utah

Program Intervention Budgets — 2014

Recommended Annual Investment	**$19.3 million**
Deaths in State Caused by Smoking	
Annual average smoking-attributable deaths	1,200
Youth aged 0-17 projected to die from smoking	38,600
Annual Costs Incurred in State from Smoking	
Total medical	$542 million
State Revenue from Tobacco Sales and Settlement	
FY 2012 tobacco tax revenue	$132.0 million
FY 2012 tobacco settlement payment	$36.4 million
Total state revenue from tobacco sales and settlement	$168.4 million
Percent Tobacco Revenue to Fund at Recommended Level	**11%**

	Annual Total (Millions)		Annual Per Capita	
	Minimum	Recommended	Minimum	Recommended
I. State and Community Interventions Multiple social resources working together will have the greatest long-term population impact.	$5.8	$7.3	$2.03	$2.56
II. Mass-Reach Health Communication Interventions Media interventions work to prevent smoking initiation, promote cessation, and shape social norms.	$2.3	$3.4	$0.81	$1.19
III. Cessation Interventions Tobacco use treatment is effective and highly cost-effective.	$4.0	$6.1	$1.40	$2.14
IV. Surveillance and Evaluation Publicly funded programs should be accountable and demonstrate effectiveness.	$1.2	$1.7	$0.42	$0.59
V. Infrastructure, Administration, and Management Complex, integrated programs require experienced staff to provide fiscal management, accountability, and coordination.	$0.6	$0.8	$0.21	$0.29
TOTAL	$13.9	$19.3	$4.87	$6.77

Note: A justification for each program element and the rationale for the budget estimates are provided in Section A. The funding estimates presented are based on adjustments for changes in population and cost-of-living increases since *Best Practices — 2007* was published. The actual funding required for implementing programs will vary depending on state characteristics, such as prevalence of tobacco use, sociodemographic factors, and other factors. See Appendix E for data sources on deaths, costs, revenue, and state-specific factors.

Centers for Disease Control and Prevention • Office on Smoking and Health
www.cdc.gov/tobacco • tobaccoinfo@cdc.gov • 1 (800) CDC-INFO or 1 (800) 232-4636

Section C: Recommended Funding Levels, by State — **Best Practices** for Comprehensive Tobacco Control Programs

Vermont

Program Intervention Budgets — 2014

Recommended Annual Investment	$8.4 million
Deaths in State Caused by Smoking	
Annual average smoking-attributable deaths	900
Youth aged 0-17 projected to die from smoking	10,100
Annual Costs Incurred in State from Smoking	
Total medical	$348 million
State Revenue from Tobacco Sales and Settlement	
FY 2012 tobacco tax revenue	$80.1 million
FY 2012 tobacco settlement payment	$34.5 million
Total state revenue from tobacco sales and settlement	$114.6 million
Percent Tobacco Revenue to Fund at Recommended Level	7%

	Annual Total (Millions)		Annual Per Capita	
	Minimum	Recommended	Minimum	Recommended
I. State and Community Interventions Multiple social resources working together will have the greatest long-term population impact.	$2.5	$3.1	$3.99	$4.95
II. Mass-Reach Health Communication Interventions Media interventions work to prevent smoking initiation, promote cessation, and shape social norms.	$1.1	$1.6	$1.76	$2.56
III. Cessation Interventions Tobacco use treatment is effective and highly cost-effective.	$1.7	$2.6	$2.72	$4.15
IV. Surveillance and Evaluation Publicly funded programs should be accountable and demonstrate effectiveness.	$0.5	$0.7	$0.85	$1.17
V. Infrastructure, Administration, and Management Complex, integrated programs require experienced staff to provide fiscal management, accountability, and coordination.	$0.3	$0.4	$0.42	$0.58
TOTAL	$6.1	$8.4	$9.74	$13.41

Note: A justification for each program element and the rationale for the budget estimates are provided in Section A. The funding estimates presented are based on adjustments for changes in population and cost-of-living increases since *Best Practices — 2007* was published. The actual funding required for implementing programs will vary depending on state characteristics, such as prevalence of tobacco use, sociodemographic factors, and other factors. See Appendix E for data sources on deaths, costs, revenue, and state-specific factors.

Centers for Disease Control and Prevention • Office on Smoking and Health
www.cdc.gov/tobacco • tobaccoinfo@cdc.gov • 1 (800) CDC-INFO or 1 (800) 232-4636

Best Practices for Comprehensive Tobacco Control Programs

Section C: Recommended Funding Levels, by State

Virginia

Program Intervention Budgets — 2014

Recommended Annual Investment	$91.6 million
Deaths in State Caused by Smoking	
Annual average smoking-attributable deaths	9,000
Youth aged 0-17 projected to die from smoking	150,300
Annual Costs Incurred in State from Smoking	
Total medical	$3,113 million
State Revenue from Tobacco Sales and Settlement	
FY 2012 tobacco tax revenue	$187.4 million
FY 2012 tobacco settlement payment	$117.4 million
Total state revenue from tobacco sales and settlement	$304.8 million
Percent Tobacco Revenue to Fund at Recommended Level	**30%**

	Annual Total (Millions)		Annual Per Capita	
	Minimum	Recommended	Minimum	Recommended
I. State and Community Interventions Multiple social resources working together will have the greatest long-term population impact.	$19.1	$23.8	$2.33	$2.91
II. Mass-Reach Health Communication Interventions Media interventions work to prevent smoking initiation, promote cessation, and shape social norms.	$15.4	$22.2	$1.88	$2.71
III. Cessation Interventions Tobacco use treatment is effective and highly cost-effective.	$21.0	$33.6	$2.57	$4.10
IV. Surveillance and Evaluation Publicly funded programs should be accountable and demonstrate effectiveness.	$5.6	$8.0	$0.68	$0.97
V. Infrastructure, Administration, and Management Complex, integrated programs require experienced staff to provide fiscal management, accountability, and coordination.	$2.8	$4.0	$0.34	$0.49
TOTAL	$63.9	$91.6	$7.80	$11.18

Note: A justification for each program element and the rationale for the budget estimates are provided in Section A. The funding estimates presented are based on adjustments for changes in population and cost-of-living increases since *Best Practices — 2007* was published. The actual funding required for implementing programs will vary depending on state characteristics, such as prevalence of tobacco use, sociodemographic factors, and other factors. See Appendix E for data sources on deaths, costs, revenue, and state-specific factors.

Centers for Disease Control and Prevention • Office on Smoking and Health
www.cdc.gov/tobacco • tobaccoinfo@cdc.gov • 1 (800) CDC-INFO or 1 (800) 232-4636

Section C: Recommended Funding Levels, by State — 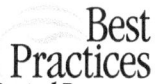 **Best Practices** for **Comprehensive Tobacco Control Programs**

Washington

Program Intervention Budgets — 2014

Recommended Annual Investment	$63.6 million
Deaths in State Caused by Smoking	
Annual average smoking-attributable deaths	7,300
Youth aged 0-17 projected to die from smoking	104,000
Annual Costs Incurred in State from Smoking	
Total medical	$2,812 million
State Revenue from Tobacco Sales and Settlement	
FY 2012 tobacco tax revenue	$471.4 million
FY 2012 tobacco settlement payment	$150.7 million
Total state revenue from tobacco sales and settlement	$622.1 million
Percent Tobacco Revenue to Fund at Recommended Level	10%

	Annual Total (Millions)		Annual Per Capita	
	Minimum	Recommended	Minimum	Recommended
I. State and Community Interventions Multiple social resources working together will have the greatest long-term population impact.	$16.4	$20.5	$2.38	$2.97
II. Mass-Reach Health Communication Interventions Media interventions work to prevent smoking initiation, promote cessation, and shape social norms.	$6.3	$9.1	$0.91	$1.32
III. Cessation Interventions Tobacco use treatment is effective and highly cost-effective.	$16.0	$25.7	$2.32	$3.73
IV. Surveillance and Evaluation Publicly funded programs should be accountable and demonstrate effectiveness.	$3.9	$5.5	$0.56	$0.80
V. Infrastructure, Administration, and Management Complex, integrated programs require experienced staff to provide fiscal management, accountability, and coordination.	$1.9	$2.8	$0.28	$0.40
TOTAL	$44.5	$63.6	$6.45	$9.22

Note: A justification for each program element and the rationale for the budget estimates are provided in Section A. The funding estimates presented are based on adjustments for changes in population and cost-of-living increases since *Best Practices—2007* was published. The actual funding required for implementing programs will vary depending on state characteristics, such as prevalence of tobacco use, sociodemographic factors, and other factors. See Appendix E for data sources on deaths, costs, revenue, and state-specific factors.

Centers for Disease Control and Prevention • Office on Smoking and Health
www.cdc.gov/tobacco • tobaccoinfo@cdc.gov • 1 (800) CDC-INFO or 1 (800) 232-4636

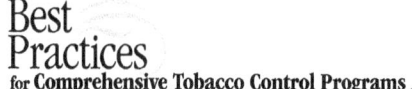

West Virginia

Program Intervention Budgets — 2014

Recommended Annual Investment	$27.4 million
Deaths in State Caused by Smoking	
Annual average smoking-attributable deaths	3,700
Youth aged 0-17 projected to die from smoking	47,300
Annual Costs Incurred in State from Smoking	
Total medical	$1,008 million
State Revenue from Tobacco Sales and Settlement	
FY 2012 tobacco tax revenue	$109.6 million
FY 2012 tobacco settlement payment	$63.7 million
Total state revenue from tobacco sales and settlement	$173.3 million
Percent Tobacco Revenue to Fund at Recommended Level	16%

	Annual Total (Millions)		Annual Per Capita	
	Minimum	Recommended	Minimum	Recommended
I. State and Community Interventions Multiple social resources working together will have the greatest long-term population impact.	$6.7	$8.4	$3.61	$4.53
II. Mass-Reach Health Communication Interventions Media interventions work to prevent smoking initiation, promote cessation, and shape social norms.	$2.6	$3.7	$1.40	$1.99
III. Cessation Interventions Tobacco use treatment is effective and highly cost-effective.	$7.4	$11.7	$3.99	$6.31
IV. Surveillance and Evaluation Publicly funded programs should be accountable and demonstrate effectiveness.	$1.7	$2.4	$0.90	$1.28
V. Infrastructure, Administration, and Management Complex, integrated programs require experienced staff to provide fiscal management, accountability, and coordination.	$0.8	$1.2	$0.45	$0.64
TOTAL	$19.2	$27.4	$10.35	$14.75

Note: A justification for each program element and the rationale for the budget estimates are provided in Section A. The funding estimates presented are based on adjustments for changes in population and cost-of-living increases since *Best Practices — 2007* was published. The actual funding required for implementing programs will vary depending on state characteristics, such as prevalence of tobacco use, sociodemographic factors, and other factors. See Appendix E for data sources on deaths, costs, revenue, and state-specific factors.

Centers for Disease Control and Prevention • Office on Smoking and Health
www.cdc.gov/tobacco • tobaccoinfo@cdc.gov • 1 (800) CDC-INFO or 1 (800) 232-4636

Section C: Recommended Funding Levels, by State — Best Practices for Comprehensive Tobacco Control Programs

Wisconsin

Program Intervention Budgets — 2014

Recommended Annual Investment	$57.5 million
Deaths in State Caused by Smoking	
Annual average smoking-attributable deaths	7,000
Youth aged 0-17 projected to die from smoking	106,200
Annual Costs Incurred in State from Smoking	
Total medical	$2,663 million
State Revenue from Tobacco Sales and Settlement	
FY 2012 tobacco tax revenue	$653.3 million
FY 2012 tobacco settlement payment	$131.1 million
Total state revenue from tobacco sales and settlement	$784.4 million
Percent Tobacco Revenue to Fund at Recommended Level	**7%**

	Annual Total (Millions)		Annual Per Capita	
	Minimum	Recommended	Minimum	Recommended
I. State and Community Interventions Multiple social resources working together will have the greatest long-term population impact.	$14.7	$18.4	$2.57	$3.21
II. Mass-Reach Health Communication Interventions Media interventions work to prevent smoking initiation, promote cessation, and shape social norms.	$4.4	$6.4	$0.77	$1.12
III. Cessation Interventions Tobacco use treatment is effective and highly cost-effective.	$15.7	$25.2	$2.74	$4.40
IV. Surveillance and Evaluation Publicly funded programs should be accountable and demonstrate effectiveness.	$3.5	$5.0	$0.61	$0.87
V. Infrastructure, Administration, and Management Complex, integrated programs require experienced staff to provide fiscal management, accountability, and coordination.	$1.7	$2.5	$0.30	$0.44
TOTAL	$40.0	$57.5	$6.99	$10.04

Note: A justification for each program element and the rationale for the budget estimates are provided in Section A. The funding estimates presented are based on adjustments for changes in population and cost-of-living increases since *Best Practices — 2007* was published. The actual funding required for implementing programs will vary depending on state characteristics, such as prevalence of tobacco use, sociodemographic factors, and other factors. See Appendix E for data sources on deaths, costs, revenue, and state-specific factors.

Centers for Disease Control and Prevention • Office on Smoking and Health
www.cdc.gov/tobacco • tobaccoinfo@cdc.gov • 1 (800) CDC-INFO or 1 (800) 232-4636

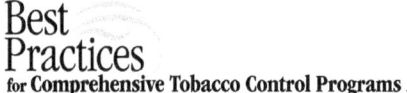

Section C: Recommended Funding Levels, by State

Wyoming

Program Intervention Budgets — 2014

Recommended Annual Investment	$8.5 million
Deaths in State Caused by Smoking	
Annual average smoking-attributable deaths	700
Youth aged 0-17 projected to die from smoking	12,100
Annual Costs Incurred in State from Smoking	
Total medical	$258 million
State Revenue from Tobacco Sales and Settlement	
FY 2012 tobacco tax revenue	$24.8 million
FY 2012 tobacco settlement payment	$18.6 million
Total state revenue from tobacco sales and settlement	$43.4 million
Percent Tobacco Revenue to Fund at Recommended Level	**20%**

	Annual Total (Millions)		Annual Per Capita	
	Minimum	Recommended	Minimum	Recommended
I. State and Community Interventions Multiple social resources working together will have the greatest long-term population impact.	$2.9	$3.6	$5.03	$6.25
II. Mass-Reach Health Communication Interventions Media interventions work to prevent smoking initiation, promote cessation, and shape social norms.	$0.6	$0.9	$1.04	$1.56
III. Cessation Interventions Tobacco use treatment is effective and highly cost-effective.	$1.9	$2.9	$3.30	$5.03
IV. Surveillance and Evaluation Publicly funded programs should be accountable and demonstrate effectiveness.	$0.5	$0.7	$0.94	$1.28
V. Infrastructure, Administration, and Management Complex, integrated programs require experienced staff to provide fiscal management, accountability, and coordination.	$0.3	$0.4	$0.47	$0.64
TOTAL	$6.2	$8.5	$10.78	$14.76

Note: A justification for each program element and the rationale for the budget estimates are provided in Section A. The funding estimates presented are based on adjustments for changes in population and cost-of-living increases since *Best Practices—2007* was published. The actual funding required for implementing programs will vary depending on state characteristics, such as prevalence of tobacco use, sociodemographic factors, and other factors. See Appendix E for data sources on deaths, costs, revenue, and state-specific factors.

Centers for Disease Control and Prevention • Office on Smoking and Health
www.cdc.gov/tobacco • tobaccoinfo@cdc.gov • 1 (800) CDC-INFO or 1 (800) 232-4636

Appendices

Appendix A: Funding Recommendation Formulations

The funding recommendations in this publication are based on the funding formulas presented in *Best Practices for Comprehensive Tobacco Control Programs—2007*. However, *Best Practices for Comprehensive Tobacco Control Programs—2014* updates the guidance provided in 2007, reflecting additional state experiences in implementing comprehensive tobacco control programs, new scientific literature, and changes in state populations, inflation, and the national tobacco control landscape since its previous release. The *recommended* levels of investment (per capita and total) are presented in 2013 dollars using 2012 population estimates. To account for inflation and changes in the U.S. population over time, these estimates can be updated using data from the U.S. Department of Labor Consumer Price Index and U.S. Census Bureau.

Best Practices for Comprehensive Tobacco Control Programs—2014 provides a streamlined two-tier funding-level framework for each state: *minimum* and *recommended*. These *minimum* and *recommended* funding levels reflect the annual investment that each state should make in order to fund and sustain a comprehensive tobacco control program. However, it is important to note that additional investments are also required at the societal level in order to most effectively reduce tobacco use.

State and Community Interventions

The budget formula and state-by-state calculations for the state and community interventions component of the report were generally based on the *Best Practices—2007* funding formulas, adjusted for population changes and inflation. However, for the 2014 update of *Best Practices*, the state and community interventions formula includes only two major components: state interventions and community interventions. The 2014 formula does not specifically include chronic disease programs to reduce the burden of tobacco-related diseases, school programs, and enforcement as major components. However, activities in these three areas may still be undertaken within the framework of state and community interventions.

Minimum and *recommended* funding levels were established for each state on the basis of the following budget items, which in turn are based on the experiences of comprehensive tobacco control programs with robust state and community programs, as previously outlined in *Best Practices—2007*.

Minimum level: The *minimum* funding level was equal to the sum of minimum statewide and community intervention costs. The minimum statewide intervention cost was equal to the total population in each state, multiplied by a variable statewide cost per person (state range: $0.58 to $1.46) that was adjusted for six state-specific factors and inflation. The minimum community intervention cost was equal to the total population in each state, multiplied by a variable community cost per person (state range: $1.02 to $1.61), adjusted for six state-specific factors and inflation, and added to a community base (state range in millions: $1.24 to $1.75).

Recommended level: The *recommended* funding level was equal to the sum of recommended statewide and community intervention costs. The recommended statewide intervention cost was equal to the minimum statewide intervention cost (which was adjusted for six state-specific factors and inflation) multiplied by a ratio of 1.25. The recommended community intervention cost was equal to the minimum community intervention cost (which was adjusted for six state-specific factors and inflation) multiplied by a ratio of 1.25.

The six state-specific factors that were used for adjustment included:

- Prevalence of smoking among adults
- Average wage rates for implementing public health programs
- The proportion of individuals within the state living at or below 200% of the poverty level

Appendix A: Funding Recommendation Formulations — **Best Practices for Comprehensive Tobacco Control Programs**

- The proportion of the population that is a racial/ethnic minority (i.e., race/ethnicity other than non-Hispanic White)
- The state's geographic size
- The state's infrastructure as reflected by the number of local governmental health units

Mass-Reach Health Communication Interventions

The budget formula and state-by-state calculations for the mass-reach health communication interventions component of the report were obtained using SQAD® 2014 cost projections for three campaign types: 1) motivating smokers to quit; 2) protecting people from the harms of secondhand smoke exposure; and 3) transforming social norms to prevent tobacco use initiation. Television media exposure was chosen because television is the primary mass-reach health communication vehicle used by most states.

Minimum level: The *minimum* level comprises delivery of an average of 1,200 GRPs per quarter for four quarters for an introductory campaign addressing either motivating smokers to quit (media buying target: adults 25–54 years of age) or protecting people from the harms of secondhand smoke exposure (media buying target: adults 25–54 years of age); and delivery of an average of 800 GRPs per quarter for four quarters for each of two ongoing campaigns: one to address transforming social norms to prevent tobacco use initiation (media buying target: youth and young adults 12–24 years of age) and one to address the campaign type not addressed in the introductory campaign (i.e. motivating smokers to quit or protecting people from the harms of secondhand smoke exposure).

Also, a 20% discount in each state's costs was made on the basis of assumed efficiencies gained from media negotiation and message synergies when three campaigns are run simultaneously. Some states receive the majority of their television exposure from stations in out-of-state markets. In these cases, a statistical approach was used to cap per capita funding at $2.16 with the assumption that media plans would be developed on the basis of cost-efficient media, such as digital.

Recommended level: The *recommended* level comprises delivery of an average of 1,600 GRPs per quarter for four quarters for an introductory campaign addressing either motivating smokers to quit (media buying target: adults 25–54 years of age) or protecting people from the harms of secondhand smoke exposure (media buying target: adults 25–54 years of age); and delivery of an average of 1,200 GRPs per quarter for four quarters for each of two ongoing campaigns: one to address transforming social norms to prevent tobacco use initiation (media buying target: youth and young adults 12–24 years of age) and one to address the campaign type not addressed in the introductory campaign (i.e. motivating smokers to quit or protecting people from the harms of secondhand smoke exposure).

Also, a 20% discount in each state's costs was made on the basis of assumed efficiencies gained from media negotiation and message synergies when three campaigns are run simultaneously. Some states receive the majority of their television exposure from stations in out-of-state markets. In these cases, a statistical approach was used to cap per capita funding at $3.10 with the assumption that media plans would be developed on the basis of cost-efficient media, such as digital.

Cessation Interventions

The budget formula and state-by-state calculations for the cessations interventions component of the report were based on four primary components: (1) promoting health systems changes; (2) providing quitline counseling; (3) providing nicotine replacement therapy through quitlines; and (4) providing cessation services via other technologies.

Minimum level: The *minimum* funding level was equal to the sum of costs associated with promoting health systems changes, providing quitline counseling, providing nicotine replacement therapy through quitlines, and providing cessation services via other technologies.

The costs of promoting health systems changes were determined using a fixed cost per state ($150,000) added to a variable cost allocated in proportion to a state's total population ($17,850,000 total). The costs of providing quitline counseling were determined using the number of quitline counseling sessions received by adult smokers per state (assumed percent of adult smokers calling quitline for assistance = 8% and percent who receive quitline counseling = 90%) multiplied by cost per call ($45.60). The costs of providing nicotine replacement therapy through quitlines were determined using the number of quitline nicotine replacement therapy treatments received by adult smokers per state (assumed percent of adult smokers calling quitline for assistance = 8%) multiplied by the estimated cost of providing 2 weeks of quitline nicotine replacement therapy ($38.00). The costs of providing cessation services via other technologies were set at a fixed value of $135,000 per state.

Recommended level: The *recommended* funding level was equal to the sum of costs associated with promoting health systems changes, providing quitline counseling, providing nicotine replacement therapy through quitlines, and providing cessation services via other technologies.

The costs of promoting health systems changes were determined using a fixed cost per state ($150,000) added to a variable cost allocated in proportion to a state's total population ($17,850,000 total). The costs of providing quitline counseling were determined using the number of quitline counseling sessions received by adult smokers per state (assumed percent of adult smokers calling quitline for assistance = 13% and percent who receive quitline counseling = 90%) multiplied by cost per call ($45.60). The costs of providing nicotine replacement therapy through quitlines were determined using the number of quitline nicotine replacement therapy treatments received by adult smokers per state (assumed percent of adult smokers calling quitline for assistance = 13%) multiplied by the estimated cost of providing 2 weeks of quitline nicotine replacement therapy ($38.00). The costs of providing cessation services via other technologies were set at a fixed value of $135,000 per state.

Surveillance and Evaluation

The budget formula and state-by-state calculations for the surveillance and evaluation component of the report were obtained by calculating 10% of the combined funding recommendation for state and community interventions, mass-reach health communication interventions, and cessation interventions in each state.

Infrastructure, Administration, and Management

The budget formula and state-by-state calculations for the infrastructure, administration and management component of the report were obtained by calculating 5% of the combined funding recommendation for state and community interventions, mass-reach health communication interventions, and cessation interventions in each state.

Appendix B:
Program and Policy Recommendations for Comprehensive Tobacco Control Programs

Guide to Community Preventive Services: What Works to Promote Health?

The Task Force on Community Preventive Service's report, *The Guide to Community Preventive Services: What Works to Promote Health?*, provides a list of effective tobacco prevention and control interventions that states and communities can implement to reduce tobacco use and exposure to secondhand smoke.[1] Tobacco control programs and their partners can compare their existing activities with these recommendations, take steps to ensure that these interventions are adequately implemented and funded, and consider additional interventions, with the ultimate goal of building and sustaining a comprehensive tobacco control program.

On the basis of evidence of effectiveness documented in the scientific literature, the Task Force's report supports the following population-based tobacco prevention and control interventions.

Population-Based Tobacco Prevention and Control Interventions

- Clean indoor air legislation prohibiting tobacco use in indoor public and private workplaces.
- Federal, state, and local efforts to increase tobacco product excise taxes as an effective public health intervention to promote tobacco use cessation and to reduce the initiation of tobacco use among youth.
- Funding and implementing long-term, high-intensity, mass-media campaigns using paid broadcast times and media messages developed through formative research.
- Proactive telephone cessation support services (quitlines).
- Reduced or eliminated copayments for effective cessation therapies.
- Reminder systems for health care providers.
- Combinations of efforts to mobilize communities to identify and reduce the commercial availability of tobacco products to youth.

The recommendations from the Task Force confirm the importance of coordinated or combined interventions for tobacco control and prevention. The evidence supporting the effectiveness of efforts to reduce tobacco use among youth through access restrictions, to institute mass-reach health communication campaigns, and to assist tobacco users to quit via telephone quitlines comes primarily from studies that implemented these interventions in combination with other strategies.

Healthy People 2020

The *Healthy People* initiative provides science-based, national objectives for improving the health of all Americans.[2] For three decades, *Healthy People* has established benchmarks and monitored progress over time in order to encourage collaborations across communities and sectors, empower individuals toward making informed health decisions, and measure the impact of prevention activities.

Healthy People 2020 was launched in 2010 and includes an ambitious, yet achievable, 10-year agenda for improving the nation's health. The national health objectives related to tobacco prevention and control are noted below.[3]

Tobacco Use

- TU-1 — Reduce tobacco use by adults.
- TU-2 — Reduce tobacco use by adolescents.
- TU-3 — Reduce the initiation of tobacco use among children, adolescents, and young adults.
- TU-4 — Increase smoking cessation attempts by adult smokers.
- TU-5 — Increase recent smoking cessation success by adult smokers.
- TU-6 — Increase smoking cessation during pregnancy.
- TU-7 — Increase smoking cessation attempts by adolescent smokers.

Health Systems Change

- TU-8 — Increase comprehensive Medicaid insurance coverage of evidence-based treatment for nicotine dependency in states and the District of Columbia.
- TU-9 — Increase tobacco screening in health care settings.
- TU-10 — Increase tobacco cessation counseling in health care settings.

Social and Environmental Changes

- TU-11 — Reduce the proportion of nonsmokers exposed to secondhand smoke.
- TU-12 — Increase the proportion of persons covered by indoor worksite policies that prohibit smoking.
- TU-13 — Establish laws in states, the District of Columbia, territories, and tribes on smokefree indoor air that prohibit smoking in public places and worksites.
- TU-14 — Increase the proportion of smokefree homes.
- TU-15 — Increase tobacco-free environments in schools, including all school facilities, property, vehicles, and school events.
- TU-16 — Eliminate state laws that preempt stronger local tobacco control laws.
- TU-17 — Increase the Federal and State tax on tobacco products.
- TU-18 — Reduce the proportion of adolescents and young adults in grades 6–12 who are exposed to tobacco marketing.
- TU-19 — Reduce the illegal sales rate to minors through enforcement of laws prohibiting the sale of tobacco products to minors.
- TU-20 — (Developmental) Increase the number of states and the District of Columbia, territories, and tribes with sustainable and comprehensive evidence-based tobacco control programs.

References

1. Zaza S, Briss PA, Harris KW, editors. *The Guide to Community Preventive Services: What Works to Promote Health?* New York: Oxford University Press, 2005.

2. U.S. Department of Health and Human Services. About Healthy People; <http://www.healthypeople.gov/2020/about/default.aspx>; accessed: December 2, 2013.

3. U.S. Department of Health and Human Services. Healthy People 2020 Objectives; <http://www.healthypeople.gov/2020/topicsobjectives2020/default.aspx>; accessed December 2, 2013.

Appendix C: National Prevention Strategy Recommendations

(National Prevention Council[1])

National Prevention Strategy Recommendations

- Support comprehensive tobacco-free and other evidence-based tobacco control policies.
- Support full implementation of the 2009 Family Smoking Prevention and Tobacco Control Act.
- Expand use of tobacco cessation services.
- Use media to educate and encourage people to live tobacco-free.

National Prevention Strategy Federal Actions	National Prevention Council Department Actions
Support states, tribes, and communities to implement tobacco control interventions and policies.	■ HHS will continue to enforce tobacco advertising and youth promotion restrictions as well as work with states to enforce age compliance checks. ■ HHS will continue to support states, tribes, and communities through the National Tobacco Control Program, which works to prevent initiation, promote quitting, eliminate disparities among population groups, and eliminate exposure to secondhand smoke through population-based community interventions, countermarketing, and data collection. ■ HUD is partnering with HHS to encourage the adoption and implementation of smoke free multi-unit housing policies among Public Housing Agencies by developing toolkits with information about smoke free living and identifying and disseminating best practices in the creation of smoke free housing.
Promote comprehensive tobacco-free worksite, campus, and conference/meeting policies.	■ DOD will implement a comprehensive tobacco control program with special emphasis on environmental and primary prevention activities to promote health and mission readiness and to lead by example. ■ DOD is working to reduce tobacco use on DOD installations to promote health and mission readiness, help tobacco users to abstain/quit, and lead by example for all workplaces.
Promote utilization of smoking cessation benefits by federal employees, Medicare and Medicaid beneficiaries, and active duty and military retirees.	■ HHS will launch a tobacco Web site that provides users with a single source of information on how to access available cessation resources to increase the use of such resources.

CONTINUED

Appendix C: National Prevention Strategy Recommendations — **Best Practices for Comprehensive Tobacco Control Programs**

National Prevention Strategy Federal Actions	National Prevention Council Department Actions
Make cessation services more accessible and available by implementing applicable provisions of the Affordable Care Act, including in government health care delivery sites.	■ HHS is working with partners to implement the expanded tobacco screening and cessation services now covered under the Affordable Care Act, including screening and cessation interventions for adults, expanded counseling for pregnant tobacco users, and full coverage for tobacco cessation services for pregnant women in states' Medicaid programs. ■ HHS will continue to match 50% of the states' cost of providing tobacco cessation telephone quitline services for Medicaid patients to support convenient delivery of such services and maximize successful tobacco cessation rates. ■ VA will support the delivery of evidence-based, effective tobacco cessation counseling to tobacco users through training health care providers, screening patients for tobacco use, offering a variety of cessation services, and monitoring tobacco cessation processes to encourage and support smoking cessation efforts of veterans who use tobacco products.
Implement the warning mandated to appear on cigarette packages and in cigarette advertisements to include new textual warning statements and color graphics depicting the negative health consequences of tobacco use, as required by FSPTCA.*	■ HHS announced the final rules requiring larger, more prominent cigarette health warning labels with accompanying color graphics in June 2011. *The FDA's final rule on cigarette graphic warnings that was required under the FSPTCA was found unconstitutional on first amendment grounds. The US Court of Appeals remanded the matter to FDA, which will undertake research to support a new rulemaking consistent with the FSPTCA.*
Research tobacco use and the effectiveness of tobacco control interventions.	■ DOD will consider how the availability of tobacco in military exchanges is contributing to tobacco consumption and how strategies outlined in *Best Practices for Comprehensive Tobacco Control Programs* can improve the health of Military Health System beneficiaries and the civilian workforce.
Encourage clinicians and health care facilities to record smoking status for patients aged 13 years or older and to report on the clinical quality measure for smoking cessation counseling, in accordance with the Medicare and Medicaid Electronic Health Records Incentive Program.	■ HHS will continue to include measures in its quality reporting programs that promote the assessment and treatment of smoking in adolescents and adults.

Abbreviations:

DOD: Department of Defense
FDA: Food and Drug Administration
FSPTCA: Family Smoking Prevention and Tobacco Control Act
HHS: Department of Health and Human Services
HUD: Department of Housing and Urban Development
VA: Department of Veterans Affairs

Reference

1. National Prevention Council. National Prevention Council Action Plan: Implementing the National Prevention Strategy; < http://www.surgeongeneral.gov/initiatives/prevention/2012-npc-action-plan.pdf >; accessed: December 2, 2013.

Appendix D: Guidelines for Comprehensive Local Tobacco Control Programs

(National Association of County and City Health Officials[1])

1. Community Interventions: $3.99 to $6.75 per person, per year

For meaningful change to occur in the way tobacco products are marketed, sold, and used, community involvement is essential. For example, promoting smokefree environments and enforcing policies that restrict tobacco advertising help to change social norms about tobacco use. Raising taxes on tobacco is among the most effective ways to reduce use, especially among young people and the poor. Restricting access to tobacco products discourages youth from initiating tobacco use, and with the new Food and Drug Administration legislation, localities will have more opportunity to influence where, when, and how tobacco products are displayed and sold.

2. Health Communications: $0.65 to $1.95 per person, per year

There is considerable evidence that communication campaigns are effective at reducing tobacco consumption. A well-coordinated mass-media campaign that reaches a wide market and warns individuals about the dangers of tobacco use can promote cessation and prevent initiation in the general population and hard-to-reach groups. Media messages can have a powerful influence on public support for tobacco control policies and help reinforce school and community efforts.

3. Cessation Interventions: $2.04 to $5.94 per adult, per year

More than two-thirds of adult smokers report a desire to quit. Cessation interventions offer the quickest and largest short-term public health benefit compared with any other component of the comprehensive tobacco control program. Many effective treatments for tobacco dependence now exist but are underused. Health care systems must better identify, treat, and refer patients addicted to tobacco use.

4. Program Administration and Management: The larger of 5% of program budget or one-quarter to one full-time equivalent (FTE) dedicated staff

Each local health department requires dedicated personnel who can perform strategic planning, staffing, and fiscal management functions, and a well-trained work force that has the skills required to carry out program activities. For even the smallest of populations, at least one-quarter full-time equivalent (FTE) staff member should be dedicated to tobacco control programming and oversight and can also serve as chronic disease lead. As the size of the population and the program increases, staff resources beyond one FTE to implement tobacco interventions should be derived from the recommended budgets of the other program components.

5. Surveillance and Evaluation: 10% of program budget

Surveillance and evaluation are essential elements of a comprehensive tobacco control program. A successful program should assess the use of tobacco, local factors contributing to tobacco use, and progress toward planned outcomes and should report data that are useful to policymakers and the public.

Reference

1. National Association of County & City Health Officials. 2010 Program and Funding Guidelines for Local Comprehensive Tobacco Control Program; <http://www.naccho.org/toolbox/tool.cfm?id=1994>; accessed: December 2, 2013.

Appendix E: Data Sources

Deaths Caused by Smoking

Annual Average Smoking-Attributable Deaths: Data were obtained from the Adult Smoking-Attributable Mortality, Morbidity, and Economic Costs (SAMMEC) system.[1] Data are annual averages among adults aged 35 years and older from 2005–2009. These estimates do not include deaths related to burns or secondhand smoke. All figures were rounded to the nearest hundred.[2]

Youth Projected to Die from Smoking: This measure is calculated using estimates of youth projected to start smoking as well as estimates of premature deaths attributable to smoking among continuing smokers and among those who quit after 35 years of age.[2] Data on the number of youth projected to start smoking were obtained using the number of persons aged 0–17 years in each state from the U.S. Census Bureau (July 1, 2012 estimates).[3] The average prevalence of smoking among adults aged 18–30 years for each state was obtained from the 2011–2012 Behavioral Risk Factor Surveillance System.[4] Data on premature deaths attributable to smoking were obtained from the Adult Smoking-Attributable Mortality, Morbidity, and Economic Costs (SAMMEC) system.[1] All figures were rounded to the nearest hundred.

Annual Costs Incurred from Smoking

Annual Costs Incurred from Smoking: Estimates were obtained on the basis of smoking-attributable fractions obtained from the Smoking-Attributable Mortality, Morbidity, and Economic Costs (SAMMEC) system,[1] and state-specific health care expenditure data were obtained from the Centers for Medicare and Medicaid Services.[5] All figures were rounded to the nearest million.

State Revenue from Tobacco Sales and Settlement

Tobacco Tax Revenue: Data for fiscal year 2012 were obtained from The *Tax Burden on Tobacco, 2012.*[6] Figures were rounded to the nearest hundred thousand.

Tobacco Settlement Payment: Data for fiscal year 2012 were obtained from the State Tobacco Activities Tracking and Evaluation (STATE) System.[7] Data were provided to the STATE System by the National Association of Attorneys General for the 46 states and District of Columbia that participated in the Master Settlement Agreement (MSA). Payments for four non-MSA states were obtained by direct contact with those states. All figures were rounded to the nearest hundred thousand.

State Revenue from Tobacco Sales and Settlement: Total figures were obtained by adding the total tobacco tax revenue and tobacco settlement payment figures above. All figures were rounded to the nearest hundred thousand.

State-Specific Factors Used in Funding Recommendation Formulas

Total Population Size, Population of Adults Aged 18 years and Older, and Population Estimates by Race: Data were obtained from the U.S. Census Bureau for total state populations (July 1, 2012 estimates).[3] The estimates are based on the 2010 Census and reflect changes to the April 1, 2010 population due to the Count Question Resolution program and geographic program revisions.

Cigarette Smoking Prevalence: Data were obtained from the 2012 Behavioral Risk Factor Surveillance System (BRFSS).[4]

Poverty Status: Data were obtained from the 2012 Annual Social and Economic Supplement (ASEC) of the Current Population Survey (CPS).[8]

Average Annual Salary to Implement Public Health Programs: Data were obtained from the 2012 Quarterly Census of Employment and Wages, U.S. Bureau of Labor Statistics.[9]

Number of Local Health Units: Data were obtained from the National Association of County and City Health Officials.[10]

Designated Market Area Cost and Reach of Targeted Audience: Data for the year 2013 were obtained from AC Nielsen through PlowShare Group Inc.[11]

Land Area: Data were obtained from the 2010 State Area Measurements and Internal Point Coordinates report of the U.S. Census Bureau.[12]

Consumer Price Index: Data were obtained from the U.S. Bureau of Labor Statistics.[13]

References

1. Centers for Disease Control and Prevention. Smoking-Attributable Mortality, Morbidity, and Economic Costs (SAMMEC); <http://apps.nccd.cdc.gov/sammec/>; accessed: December 2, 2013.

2. Centers for Disease Control and Prevention. Smoking-Attributable Mortality, Years of Potential Life Lost, and Productivity Losses — United States, 2000–2004. *Morbidity and Mortality Weekly Report.* 2008;57(45):1226–8.

3. U.S. Census Bureau. Population Estimates; <http://www.census.gov/>; accessed: December 2, 2013.

4. Centers for Disease Control and Prevention. Behavioral Risk Factor Surveillance System; <http://www.cdc.gov/brfss/>; accessed: December 2, 2013.

5. Centers for Medicaid and Medicare Services. National Health Expenditure Date; <http://www.cms.gov/Research-Statistics-Data-and-Systems/Statistics-Trends-and-Reports/NationalHealthExpendData/index.html>; accessed: December 2, 2013.

6. Orzechowski W, Walker RC. *The Tax Burden on Tobacco,* 2012. Tables 9, 12, and 19. Arlington, VA: Orzechowski and Walker, 2013.

7. Centers for Disease Control and Prevention. State Tobacco Activities Tracking and Evaluation (STATE) System; <http://www.cdc.gov/tobacco/statesystem>; accessed: December 2, 2013.

8. U.S. Census Bureau. Annual Social and Economic Supplement (ASEC) of the Current Population Survey (CPS); <http://www.census.gov/cps/data/cpstablecreator.html>; accessed: December 2, 2013.

9. United States Department of Labor. Quarterly Census of Employment and Wages; <http://data.bls.gov/>; accessed: December 2, 2013.

10. National Association of County and City Health Officials. Local Health Units, by State. Unpublished data. 2012.

11. PlowShare Group Inc. Unpublished data. 2013.

12. U.S. Census Bureau. State Area Measurements and Internal Point Coordinates; <http://www.census.gov/geo/reference/state-area.html>; accessed: December 2, 2013.

13. U.S. Department of Labor. Consumer Price Index; <http://www.bls.gov/cpi/tables.htm>; accessed: December 2, 2013.

Notes:

Notes:

www.ingramcontent.com/pod-product-compliance
Lightning Source LLC
Chambersburg PA
CBHW081726170526
45167CB00009B/3714